To all women in the world
judgment, afraid of not being heard
but who want to achieve more, want to break the glass ceiling, want to have an impact in their own world and feel liberated from self-imposed limitations. This book is for all women who want to unlock their true essence and skyrocket their lives and dreams!

Stop Believing The B.S.!

7 Steps to Awaken Your ***Feminine Power***

Eva Martins

Stop the B.S.!
7 Steps to Awaken Your Feminine Power

ISBN 9798682694044

The strategies in this book are presented for educational purposes. All quotes remain the proprietary property of the authors. Every effort has been made to trace copyright holders and obtain permission for the use of copyrights material where applicable.

The information and resources presented are based on the author's personal experience and opinion. Any outcome or results vary with each individual. There is no guarantee as to the results.

The author reserves all rights to make changes and assumes no responsibility or liability on behalf of any purchaser, reader or user of these materials.

For complimentary templates and workbooks to accompany the 7 transformational Steps to Awaken Your Feminine Power in this book, while available, visit www.evamartins.com .

First Edition

Acknowledgements

Writing this book has been an amazing and transformational journey I started many years ago. It is my tribute to women, to the feminine energy. I wrote this book to inspire and encourage women to embrace their authentic being with all its gifts and power.

I did struggle as many other women, rejecting my own voice, my own wishes, my own strengths as a way to belong, sacrificing my happiness for others. The universe always had my back and gifted my life with beautiful souls who showed be the example, who inspired me, who supported me beyond my expectations…

Thank you to my mum Edith, for being the most inspiring example of feminine power in my life. You always went for your dreams, defied the norms, showing the example to many women that we could be independent emotionally and professionally, not allowing your fears to stop you. Showing me that I could be strong, independent, and that I could achieve everything. Thank you for always being there, in the beautiful moments but also during the difficult periods of our life. I know I might not express it often, but I am really grateful, and I love you deeply. Thank you for inspiring me.

Thank you to my dad Manuel, for inspiring me to take risks in life, for showing me that my deepest dreams could become a reality, for inspiring my manifesting powers, for the creativity and innovative mindset I inherited from you. Thank you for your constant love and emotional support, your words might not express a lot, but your eyes speak for them. I love you deeply even though I might have not said it enough…

Thank you to my brother Philippe, for constantly testing me, for showing me my power, for trusting me, for accepting me as I am, for being there when I need, for forcing me to step up, for always speaking your truth, for being a strong pillar in my life. I know you are always there for me, same as I do. I am grateful you are in my life, even when you challenge me, love you bro…

Thank you to my soul mate Beren, for all your unconditional love, for your constant emotional support. With you I discovered a new dimension in life, filled with unconditional love, deep connection, common dreams and values, real partnership, beautiful growth, caring and fun. I can't foresee my life without you…Your dedication to fulfill me, to make me happy on the day to day allowed me to open my wings, to embrace this new challenge and write this book…without you I would have never had the courage. I love you deeply. Love is only a word until someone gives it a meaning …YOU. Thank you for accepting my dedication to growth and somehow my beautiful craziness. A lifelong partner, lover, husband, friend making both the journey and destination magical.

Thank you to my beautiful daughters Catherine and Caroline, for being the most beautiful souls I ever had the chance to meet. It is a privilege to be your mum. Your unconditional love, your daily caring has allowed me to heal deeply and uncover what unconditional love is. Your power, your compassion, your values, your love, your smartness, your dedication to make the world a better place have been inspiring me every day. I have embraced my courage and wrote this book to show you that we should always go for our dreams independently of others feedback, following our own inner truth and not play small in life otherwise we betray our own dreams…

Thank you to my beautiful son Thomas. I love your little happy soul, bringing light and fun to our day to day. You have so much love to give, you are such a sensitive soul that you will make any woman the happiest on earth. Your smartness and curiosity inspire me every day to go deeper in my knowledge, they always trigger new thoughts, new dimensions. You have been a beautiful gift from the universe. The one thing I am the most grateful for is how you teach me acceptance at the deepest level, accepting of what it is, accepting that we are all different and it is perfect, showing me that there are always many different ways and it is ok, showing me how to step up in my unconditional love.

Thank you to the universe for gifting my life with amazing souls. Thank you to Ana, for always being there, to laugh, to cry, to create, to grow, to have fun…. without you some of the moments of my life would have been much darker and some others less bright. Thank you for inspiring me, for being a wonderful example of what feminine power is, for your love, for your caring, for kicking me when I need it. Thank you for accepting me in your life as your Sis!

And finally thank you to all the amazing women I met in my life who inspired me. Thank you to Yasmin for igniting my spiritual life. Thank you, Marie, for always being there, for your love, for your acceptance and unconditional support. Thank you, Joana and Ana L, for being part of my journey, for listening to me, for comforting me when I needed it the most, for your love. Thank you, Suzi, for bring me my soul mate...Thank you to Mathilde for being a beautiful bonus daughter, for your support, love and for being a beautiful soul.

Thank you!
Eva

7 steps to Awaken Your Feminine Power

1 – Letting go of the Masks

2 – Understanding the Whys

3 – Uncovering the Truth

4 – Understand the Pain

5 – Going Deeper

6 – Taking Action

7 – Being Inspired

Just embrace the journey to uncover your feminine radiance …

Table of Contents

Introduction

- Are you trying to be perfect in all areas of your life, but feeling unhappy?
- Are you a corporate woman or entrepreneur trying hard to be successful and independent financially?
- Are you constantly competing with men, or other women, just trying to be heard?
- Do you think you need to be stronger, more masculine to be successful in your career?
- Are you pushing away your true emotions just to be taken seriously?

If you replied yes to any of these questions, this book is for you!

All of my life I have rejected my true feminine power until I understood its true nature. Once I understood that I was disconnecting with myself, my true self, everything changed. I understood that the more I was pushing my power away, the more I was pushing away money, love, happiness, true relationships, fulfillment, feeling connected with life. I was voluntarily being a passenger instead of being in the driver seat of my own life.

I had to go through a self-discovery journey, lessons, challenges to understand its true origins, identity, force, sensitivity and power. I took a journey to understand the feminine and masculine potential in each other, in ourselves, how they complement one another and how they can uplift and empower each other instead of annihilating each other.

Being a strong corporate woman, a leader, a mother, a wife, a daughter, a friend, and every other role you fulfill is extremely challenging nowadays. I understand. It's exhausting trying to be perfect in all areas of life: being a sensitive, receptive and guiding mother, empowering our children to be independent kids while keeping them safe; being a nice, caring and sexy wife; and being a go-getter at work. I, for one, felt like I was sacrificing myself almost all of the time.

The environment is demanding, and you feel you need to be at your best every day.

I felt this way too. And I almost lost myself along the way....

Born in Paris, in a feministic country where women are encouraged to be strong, vocal, and independent in a family where the mother was the leader, the strong voice, I learned that this was how to be the authority. I copied a model that equated "successful" with this strong force, having clear objectives and going for it no matter what the cost. It became a survival need in order to fit in.

I started my career in a male-dominated corporate industry where you soon understand that if you do not have power, you go nowhere. And how did you get power? Your ideas had to be heard. But the few women in my office and I, experienced that if you do not have a strong voice, you are not heard. That is, if you do not adopt a more masculine attitude you were blocked from exceling.

If we showed our passion and feminine drive, we were seen as too emotional. So, we numbed ourselves, rejected our intuition and sensitive side and allowed our masculine energy and assertiveness to take over. But without balance, most of the time it was too much. So, we were seen as being highly demanding and extremely competitive, even towards each other. Does any of this sound familiar?

It took me more than 10 years of operating in many different leading roles to realize what was happening. I had a successful career, but I was sacrificing myself, disconnecting from who I was and actually limiting my full potential.

I will never forget the day I woke up and felt that I had no more feelings. There was no feeling of connection anymore. I was doing more and more every day and it was never enough. Everything was a struggle.

Doing my best at work and feeling exhausted, coming back home to pick up the kids, play with them, giving them a bath, preparing the dinner, reading stories to allow them to fall asleep and feeling more and more alone and sad inside of myself…not being able to express it, not feeling understood, not feeling heard either…and all of this with constant arguments that it was not enough, having to be a beautiful, smiley wife and always ready for him… I was there for everyone… except myself.

My light was slowly vanishing. The universe pushed me so hard that I had to wake up…or extinguish my soul.

I started a new journey of conscious self-discovery, uncovering mind programs, patterns and beliefs which were limiting instead of empowering me. I began to understand the misconceptions of the feminine and masculine powers.

Living and embodying our feminine self-identity, with all its beauty and sensitivity, is in fact much more powerful and fulfilling than always being in masculine energy. In our feminine energy, we can still be this strong force of nature, taking action and moving forward.

I would love to share with you how to avoid the same mistakes, pretending being something you're not, rejecting your own inner self.

I will help you uncover your own feminine gifts and how you can experience them fully!

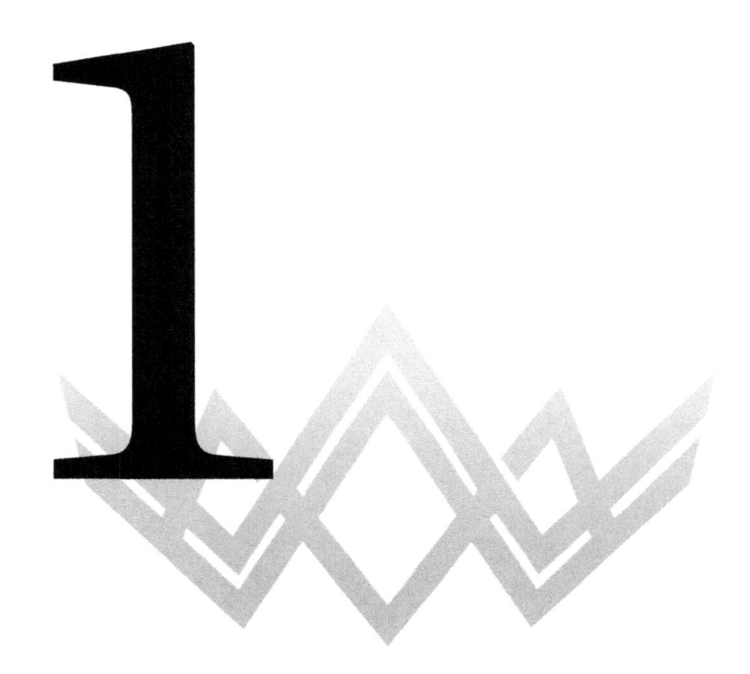

1 Letting go of the Masks

What's the Truth of the Feminine Power and Radiance?

First you need to know that there is nothing wrong in being feminine, in having emotions, in being sensitive in cultivating your feminine radiance.

Being a woman is to be a creation of many factors, going far beyond the physiological. I have studied this for many years in myself and others, spending more than a decade trying to find my feminine energy and its true identity. I have dedicated the last few years cultivating it, loving it, and teaching it to others.

Here is what I found to be true for me:

Feminine radiance is FEELING, SENSITIVITY, OPENNESS, EMPATHY, LOVING, INTUITION, NURTURING, CARING, COMPASSION.

It's not about our body type, our sexuality, our hair style, or how we dress up. It is entirely about our inner self, our energy and how we project in life. Men and women have a feminine energy and the secret is in the balance of this with our masculine energy.

A man or a woman rejecting their feminine energy may replace the emptiness, rejected emotions, missing softness and intuition by a strong sense of achievement, by a need to protect themselves, shielded from deeper loving emotions, striving for accomplishment. There is a disconnect between the heart and the mind, letting the mind govern their life. There is a need to be successful to survive. A need to be safe and protected, supported by an unconscious lack of trust preventing them from fully opening.

Feminine radiance is CREATION and INTELLIGENCE. It is the creative force of life.

The feminine energy is always feeling and sensing everything, processing everything at once, multitasking. The left and right brain are constantly active and ingesting information, which is extremely powerful. In contrast, the masculine energy is focused on one task at the time.

The feminine is about **being** while the masculine is about **doing**.

Over the years, we were all trained, men and women alike, to reject our feminine energy. In misunderstanding its openness, sensitivity, empathy to weakness, we thought we had to reject our emotions to be strong. But actually, it takes courage to be truly open. It takes strength to be in the truth and speaking the truth.

Feminine energy needs to feel safe and protected. When feeling unsafe, unseen, not understood, the feminine energy numbs itself, putting on a masculine mask. Being action driven, numbing its emotions, being competitive and fighting for survival is the default.

Masculine energy needs appreciation. It needs to feel admired and praised. When a masculine energy is feeling criticized, controlled or feeling closed off, it shifts into wearing the feminine mask.

The secret is in balancing both within ourselves to unlock real freedom, joy and happiness. Let's look at the average relationship. In order for there to be attraction, one person has to be primarily in their masculine and the other person in their feminine, like magnets attracting each other. So, imagine being a woman and constantly being in your masculine.

What do you think it does to your intimate relationship? How do you think you relate with your husband, by being action driven and numbing your emotions?

Over time, it kills any attraction and deeper connection. It's the same for men. If in stress, you go to your feminine energy and stay there for a long period of time, no longer making decisions and taking action, the same happens. Any polarity that has attracted you falls away and with time you disconnect with your true identity of your soul and it will reflect in every area of your life, starting with your love relationships.

For years it was believed that men and women's brains were wired differently, as stated in the book Men are from Mars, and Women are from Venus. We erroneously believed that men had a masculine energy and women had feminine energy. But those are just two archetypes. Research shows that neurologically we are a mosaic of both traits, showcasing one or the other depending on the situation and area of our life.

The latest research, conducted by Daphna Joel, a professor of neuroscience at Tel Aviv University failed to find consistent differences in the brain scans of more than 1400 men and women. She found that we are a beautiful mixture of both traits. As she describes in her article, only less than 8% were representing the archetype of only one or the other. The vast majority were somewhere in the middle, showing that the gender isn't binary. We are all a blend.

I have created a test that I use with my clients in order to help them understand which is their core (natural primary energy) and to determine if they are habitually more in their feminine or masculine. It is an interesting way to understand where we can refocus to be in symbiose with our core.

You can also take the test for free online on my website www.evamartins.com

Test: Which is your core? Do you have more feminine energy or masculine energy?

Read each statement and just select whichever fits the best for you, 'a' or 'b'. Then count how many 'a's and how many 'b's you've chosen.

My future is
a. I am open to life's surprises, opportunities and to make the most of it as it brings zest into my life. I am willing to change course if needed.
b. I am focused on my long-term plan and on my commitments – I am very trustworthy. I do what I say I will do without changing my mind or getting distracted.
I am
a. I am pragmatic and effective. I tend to be focused, direct, and results-focused.

b. I am supportive, caring, sensual and I love beautiful adornments.
Change for me is
a. Change is part of life. I am comfortable with change and even enjoy it.
b. Schedules and routines allow me to be productive and achieve my goals. I feel uncomfortable when people change plans at the last minute.
At work
a. I enjoy collaborating with my colleagues - discussing projects and meeting my deadlines, all at the same time.
b. I prefer being focused on what I need to do to meet my deadline and commitments without the distractions of other people.
What motivates me
a. My mission is to contribute to a better world, do something bigger than myself. I adapt my goals constantly based on my mission.
b. I find my motivation through the achievement of my goals.
Going on a holiday with your partner I...
a. Let them handle most of the arrangements and look forward to the surprises ahead.

b. Plan everything beforehand so I know what we're doing.
Emotional Intensity
a. I am comfortable with the flow of life. I know how to navigate my emotions and others' emotions as well.
b. I have no patience for victimhood and emotional people. I am pragmatic and I focus on what I need to achieve.
Socially
a. I enjoy spending time with my friends and family, but I am even more fulfilled in achieving my goals.
b. I enjoy being with myself in silence, but I am more fulfilled enjoying life with my friends and family, laughing, having fun with them.
I feel best when my partner
a. Is truly listening to me and understands me.
b. Shows me that I am needed and appreciated.
My Passion is...
a. Being able to contribute to something bigger than myself.
b. Filled by a strong desire to accomplish my goals.

When taking care of a task...
a. I am a natural multitasker. I am able to speak with my partner, think about my next day and cook dinner simultaneously.
b. I am able to do many activities at the same time, but I prefer to focus my attention on one activity at a time. This is when I am at my best.

Remember, regardless of gender, we all have both masculine and feminine energy. Our core energy reflects our inner nature and values. Understanding it allows us to be aligned with ourselves and feel fulfilled – or else we will be unhappy no matter how much we succeed.

If you have more 'a's than 'b's, your leading energy is feminine.

With a leading feminine energy, you are most likely highly sensing and feeling. You are often multitasking. Your left and right part of the brain are always active, which can be extremely powerful if you are able to balance both traits. You are comfortable with your feelings and dealing with others, having a natural empathy for the emotion of others. You love being heard, seen and understood. In order to be fully opened to receive, you need to feel safe and protected.

On the other hand, if you feel unsafe, unseen or feeling misunderstood, you easily go to your masculine side. In this energy, you are often numbing your emotions, becoming more goal driven. This happens quite often in the workplace triggered by the pressure and competition.

You need to watch out in case you are triggered and go to the opposite of your core energy. Most who are feminine in their core will put on a masculine mask to protect themselves. You end up not being authentic. You end up limiting your own potential. Core feminine-energy women protect themselves by shifting more into their masculine energy. However, core masculine-energy men, when feeling insecure, protect themselves, and end up feeling insecure being more in their feminine energy.

If more 'b's than 'a's, your leading energy is masculine.

If your leading energy is masculine, you are able to be really focused and perform one task at a time. You are much more comfortable in doing, thinking, protecting, and making things happen instead of sensing, being, and feeling.

You are competitive and love achieving your goals in the timeframe you imposed on yourself. You love action and movement. You crave the sensitivity of the feminine energy which makes you feel appreciated and needed. It allows you a space to relax and connect to your heart and your emotions.

When feeling criticized, controlled and closed off, you put on a feminine mask, numbing yourself, shutting down and withdrawing. This makes the feminine energy person feel unsafe and withdraw as well.

Just as with the feminine energy at its core, if you put on the opposite mask you kill any kind of polarization in your relationship. Over time this hinders any kind of attraction and chemistry.

We find freedom, happiness, joy and fulfillment in the balance of both qualities, when we know how and when to consciously use one or the other.

Flexible	Active
Expressive	Direct
Nurturing	Ambitious
Empathic	Competitive
Free Spirit	Reliable
Creative	Rebellious
Gentle	Decisive
Intuitive	Logical

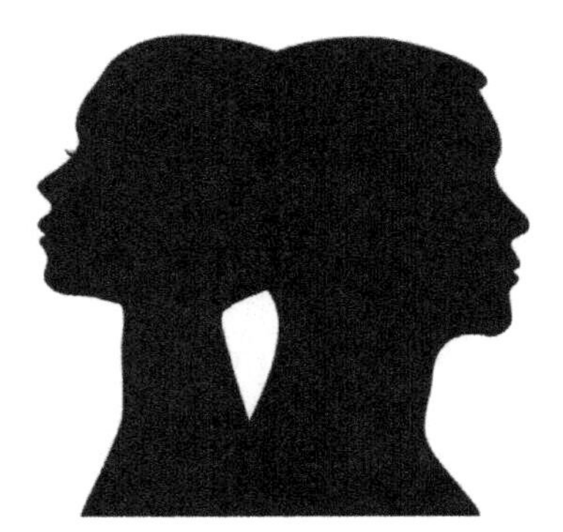

Expressing power/strength and love/caring consciously is wisdom. Men and women having feminine and masculine balanced energies are strong, caring, intuitive and wise, and generally with high emotional intelligence.

Strength is the true power of the soul when expressed with love and not "power over another". The definitions of strength and power have been misunderstood as a way to get something, to control and have a gain. True power resides in wholeness, feeling whole and complete, in feeling in love with life and oneself.

True unconditional love is a deep feeling expressed from the heart without outer motives. A high intensity of love, combined with inner power, is wisdom in its most beautiful form. It is allowing our intuition (deep inner knowing) to guide our life, words, thoughts, and actions with confidence.

The good news is that our innate nature is balanced.

What takes us out of balance is our life journey - people who have influenced us, our parents' example and expectations, experiences that have traumatized us, the collective consciousness, the environment, the culture we live in or where our parents came from, religions, relationships, the media, social medias, movies, etc.

Do You Really Know Who You Are Underneath the Masks?

We are so used to playing roles in life. We are a mother, a friend, a partner, a lover, a leader, that we forget what moves us, who we are, what we love, what we want to achieve and what we want to become in life. One day, we realize, "I do not know who I am anymore".

We hide ourselves behind the labels, following the collective consciousness or what we are supposed to be, instead of allowing our soul to burst through us.

Every day, I meet women and men trying to be something to please someone or trying to be successful following a formula instead of following their own path.

It all seems to work until one day you understand it is not your life and you start questioning all things around you. You ask yourself why you are not fulfilled. It is simply because you are negating the expression of your soul desires, negating your inner voice, your wishes, your unique identity.

If we truly believe in the power of diversity, we should not follow formulas from others - we should find our own. And by that, I do not mean abandoning any guidance, any rules. I propose to balance the choices we make, to raise our own awareness and make decisions consciously instead of following others like a zombie.

Life does not happen to us; life happens for us. We just need to understand and uncover the whys of our experiences. It does not only happen for us to grow, but also for us to learn and contribute even more to each other.

Exercise 1: An extremely powerful, simple exercise is to take a few quiet minutes for yourself. Sit straight up. Take five slow deep breaths in and out. To focus on your heart and slow your brain waves, you can put your hand on your heart. Close your eyes to better connect with your soul.

Now, simply ask yourself, "Who am I?". Keep asking and breathing, even if nothing immediately comes to mind. Then ask yourself out loud the following questions:

- "Who am I really?"
- "Who am I beyond the roles I play in life?"
- "If there was no one around me in life who would I have to be?"
- "If there was nothing I had to do, who would I want to be?"
- After each question, go deeper by asking "and *what else?*"

In listening to your responses, you'll start uncovering your true nature and what really motivates you. Write down everything that comes to mind without any kind of judgment or analysis.

Just do this simple and powerful exercise for a few minutes every day for 21 days to have more clarity on who you are and go more deeply.

In the beginning, you might uncover all the lies you have been telling yourself. This is powerful. As you continue the exercise you will go deeper and deeper to really reconnect your true identity with your soul, with your dreams and passions.

Understanding the Whys

Why Do We Reject Our True Feminine Radiance?

Finding true feminine role models is very rare.

Why is that? We want to be seen. We want to be valued. We want to be heard and acknowledged. We want to fit in and to be accepted. So, we become what we think is required to achieve this. It is how we have been socialized.

We unconsciously copy the patterns we observed from our parents, friends, society, from the collective consciousness, a set of beliefs held by the society or country we live in. It's the energy that has been all around us for centuries.

We reject our true feminine power or radiance because we are afraid of it. We may subconsciously think that having power is scary. Disempowering thoughts such as "If I have power I might use it wrongly", "If I am powerful I'll need to take care of others and I am afraid of responsibility", "If I have power I am more visible but I'm afraid of it", "Power is only for rich people", "Power is only for smart people", "I run away from power to keep hidden", "I am not powerful enough", "If I am powerful I might abuse others", "Power is bad", "Power kills".

All are stories and lies well hidden in our subconscious mind coming from thousands of years of collective consciousness. We might not even know why we act or think a certain way.

Exercise 2: Write down all of the beliefs you have around power. If you do not know consciously everything you believe, keep asking yourself *"What else is power to me?"*.

Just as in exercise 1, prepare your mind, body and heart with five deep breaths in and out, and close your eyes, while focusing on your heart. Ask yourself everything you believe is true regarding power. Once again, no judgement and analysis, just write them down. Even if you do not believe in them consciously, by writing down everything coming up in your mind, you'll access everything that your subconscious mind is unlocking for you.

- Power is...
- My power is...
- People using power are...
- After each question, go deeper by asking *"and what else?"*

When you ask yourself a question, your mind always replies. At first, the answer might not make any sense. Your role is to not judge it. Just allow it to come. You will realize most of it is nonsense, as it might be from the collective consciousness, from habit or from others. But if you uncovered it, it is because it is a belief that is running in your subconscious mind.

Most of these beliefs are thoughts we're thinking hundreds of times a day. They became our "truths", subconsciously ruling our life.

They might have been projected from our environment, our parents, our role models, our friends and family.

Most people think being powerful is having a lot, commanding others, making others do what we want without questioning it. The misconception of power comes from the inner need to take from others as a way to fill the inner emptiness and sense of lack. They just do not understand that the more they try to fill this void, the more it grows with time, and the more they are disconnecting from others.

All of those patterns of thoughts come from hundreds of years of programming through religions, societies, kingdoms, governments, communities. They are a consequence of the fear of not being valued and worthy, thinking that we are only valued for what we have, for what position we hold and for what we represent in the hierarchy of the society.

It does not need to be that way. It starts with us reclaiming who we really are. It's time to come home to ourselves.

It's time to honor the sacred feminine within ourselves - the nurturing, empathic, intuitive and compassionate side of ourselves. It's time to open up to the wisdom of who we really are. True power resides in opening up to our own vulnerability and having the courage to open deep within. Understand that we won't be able to deeply connect with others and be respected and valued if we do not do these things with ourselves first.

Emptiness never attracts anybody. So please first fill your own glass with your self-respect and self-love. Others will replicate your patterns, especially your kids, family and friends.

I am on this journey as well. I spent decades of my life rejecting the feminine for fear that I would appear soft, vulnerable, and essentially powerless, which would make me feel unsafe. I saw the feminine as weakness and I would do everything I could to feel safe. I lived in "drive-and-strive" energy for a good twenty years in organizations that relied on it, cultivated it and expected it. I tried to be the "perfect" woman, mom, wife, friend...making time for all of them and trying to be perfect as a way to be valued and loved.

I realized that I was doing this as a way to prove to myself that I was worthy of their love. All of these were misconceptions. Nothing can fill you from the outside. Things from outside are temporary - it needs to come from within.

I kept rejecting my feminine essence until the very cost of denying who I was and how I was meant to be in the world became too great. I got so disconnected with myself that I had no choice but to start out on a new journey.

It was a rocky path with some stones in the way with ups and downs. It took me a few years to really understand that the denying of my core qualities, the things that make me come alive and ignite my soul, were actually my feminine aspects that were crying out to be seen, heard and valued.

I tapped into my ability to nurture others as well as myself, my kindness, my passion, my laughter, my humor, my creativity, my intuition, my sensitivity, my positive expression and indeed, my femininity itself. I also tapped into my physical expression of my feminine power. There's nothing wrong in expressing your feminine physically. It is actually super powerful to own yourself.

Most importantly, I was rejecting my feminine power as a way to reject my true creative and intelligent power. This life force is what guides us towards what we are meant to achieve in life - our life - our purpose.

The more I was trying to be perfect the less I was, and the more I was harshly criticizing myself. Have you ever experienced this?

I did see how my masculine energy served me however. It was the fuel for my growth. Being challenge-driven, as many women, I was pushing myself to grow every day, attracting more and more challenges as a way to prove myself. But I was being less and less kind with myself as I lived more in my masculine energy.

Until one day, I could not recognize myself. I didn't know what I wanted anymore. I was numb, going through life for others…not for myself.

I was tired of proving myself. Tired of doing instead of being. Tired of giving and ending up feeling empty.

As I made few attempts to retrain my brain, I understood that there was nothing to prove. Perfection was just a myth. It was all BS! In this new consciousness, I had to change many things. But other things changed organically - friends, divorce, environment, work.

Ultimately, I had an inner awareness and consciousness of what is really important to me, and what drives real fulfillment and joy.

My new mantra became:

Life is too short to be boring,
Life is too short to be serious,
Joy and laughter enhance my power,
By loving myself I become a magnet for others,
By respecting myself others respect me...
Life happens for me and not to me!

STOP

BELIEVING THE

B.S. *OF YOUR*

MIND NOW!

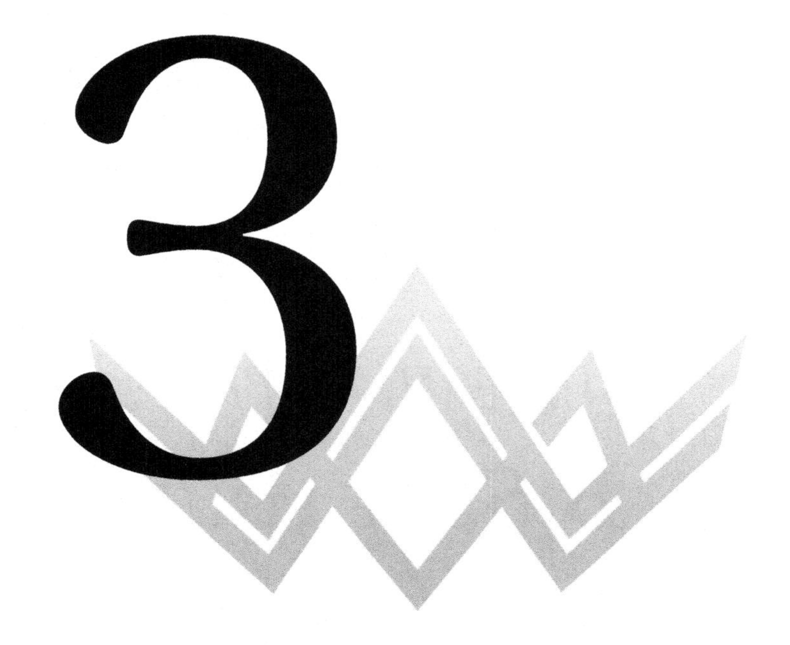

3 Uncovering the Truth

How to Identify the True Essence of Your Power?

Having worked with hundreds of women, I realized that they were rejecting their own power by misunderstanding its origin. Often thinking it meant overruling others, instead of owning themselves and their own gifts; being afraid of abusing others, afraid it would trigger big changes in their lives, afraid of being rejected, not loved, not appreciated…they often played weak as a consequence and rejected any responsibility for their own lives.

If they would know the real source of power comes from love, from respect, from non-judgement, from acceptance and gratefulness, I am sure they would embrace it. But responsibility comes by speaking up for your own truth, imposing at times your boundaries, respecting yourself first, owning your gifts and sharing them with the world.

For some it can be scarier than rejecting it. It is easier to play small than owning it, but it comes at the cost of their own fulfillment.

Exercise 3: Let's review the way you have expressed your own power during your life.

You know the drill by now. Prepare your mind, body and heart with five deep breaths in and out, close your eyes, while focusing on your heart. Ask yourself everything you believe is true regarding power. Once again, no judgement and analysis, just write them down. Even if you do not believe in them consciously, by writing down everything that is coming up in your mind, you'll access everything that your subconscious mind is unlocking for you.

Divide your life into four age segments as per the table below. In segment one, describe any moment you felt powerful, self-confident, skilled, capable of anything. Describe what happened, which skills you used, how you felt. Repeat this for the other age segments. Describe as many experiences as you can, with a minimum of 3 in each age category.

Do you recognize any patterns? Any similarities? Highlight them.

From 0 to 7 (Beginning Primary School ↓)	7 to 14 (Teenager Transition ↓)	14 to 21 (Beginning of Adult Life & Independence ↓)	Above 21
Experiences:			
Patterns:			

What have you realized? Which were the patterns you identified? Where are they coming from? Your parents? Your friends? Your Family? The environment?

And now let's start again. But this time describe any moment you felt powerless. Moments where you felt you were not enough, not capable. Describe what happened, what you felt.

Just as before, describe a minimum of three experiences in each age group and then observe and see if you are able to notice any pattern in terms of behaviors and emotions. Highlight them.

Beginning Primary School ↓ | Teenager Transition ↓ | Beginning of Adult Life & Independence ↓

From 0 to 7	7 to 14	14 to 21	Above 21
Experiences:			
Patterns:			

Any conclusions? Any patterns? Take a few moments to realize the truth behind the games you may have played unconsciously.

Bringing it to your conscious mind is the first step towards freedom. You will be able to recognize it from now on and change it consciously to retrain your thoughts, your behaviors, and consequently your beliefs. As world-renowned life coach, Tony Robbins says, *"Repetition is the mother of skills"*.

The best way to embrace your power is to get to know it, understand its values and its gifts.

In conclusion, do you know now what power means for you? We all have beliefs around power. We've uncovered a few earlier. But do you know where your real power comes from? We all have a different way of expressing it and owning it, so the best way is to ask yourself.

Exercise 4: Concluding from the previous exercise, ask yourself what power really means for me

What power means for me? How do I express my power? How would I like to express my power? In the moments where I felt powerful, how did I feel? What did I think? How did I act?

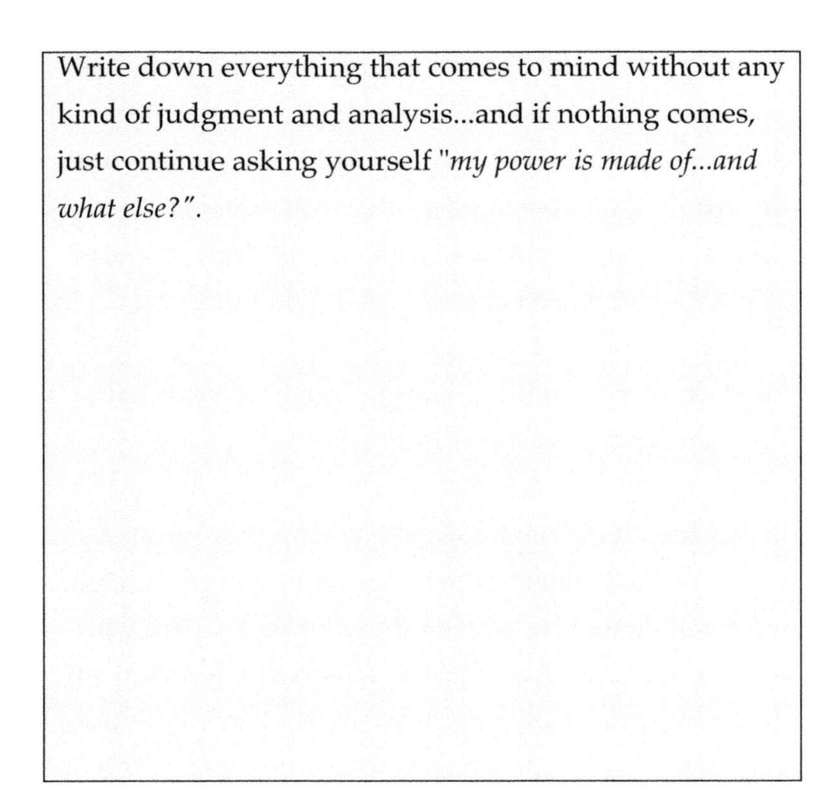

What have you uncovered? What is the truth? Take a few minutes to review your notes from the exercises above and come back to them each time you are afraid of shining in the world.

Tell yourself "If I am not sharing myself authentically, I am betraying myself and betraying others - I am negating my gifts".

4

Understand the Pain

What are the Consequences of Rejecting Your Own Feminine Power?

Rejecting our own feminine power costs big. Apart from not being authentic, and consequently feeling unhappy and unfulfilled, you are rejecting your own self, your true identity.

Does any of the following sound familiar? You slowly disconnect from your soul, your life, until you wake up and do not understand why you are there, what you are doing, or why you are living this life. You do not feel joy anymore. Laughter and happiness are gone. You are just a zombie going through life, not living it fully but pretending it is alright.

Feminine power rejection consequences also show up in your relationships. You never feel fully connected so it does not fulfill you anymore. You disconnect from both self-love and from true unconditional love with your partner/lover.

I believe we've all been there - not expressing our opinion in order to please others; not expressing our wishes but fulfilling wishes from others. Or feeling guilty or ashamed when we do put our wishes first.

How many times have you been in a meeting and felt unable to express your ideas? And after someone else expressed everything you wanted to say, they are valued for it and you feel upset with yourself. Does this sound familiar? It happened to me thousands of times. I pretended it was ok. I convinced myself that I was simply observing and listening. But the truth was that I was frustrated with myself. I allowed my fear of being judged to silence me.

Most of the time the consequences of rejecting our feminine power reflects at work. We work but are not feeling valued, recognized and fulfilled.

It also affects us financially.

Money and power are intimately linked. By rejecting your true feminine power, you also reject money abundance in all areas of your life.

How Rejecting Your Own Power Impacts Your Wealth?

Yes, rejecting your own feminine power impacts your wealth.

Since the beginning of money's existence, it has been associated with power.

The goal is not simply to finish rich, but to become the powerful force you were meant to be. Stepping in your greatness to achieve your life mission, your purpose.

Meanwhile, by rejecting your true inner power, you unconsciously reject money in your life. This is the money meant to fund your life mission and purpose!

Women's challenges with money rarely have to do with money itself, but about our fear of being powerful, of using our power.

The concept of power has been misunderstood and abused for centuries. We'd rather stay small, safe and protected than risk owning our greatness.

I would highly recommend the book from Barbara Stanny, Sacred Success – A Course in Financial Miracles. Barbara defines sacred success as *"pursuing your soul's purpose for your own bliss and the benefit of others, while being richly rewarded"*. The book allows us to better understand the relationship between power and money and how they complement each other. Both concepts of power with financial gain have been linked during thousands of years — with a special negative impact on women.

For centuries, some people have abused their authority as a way to get money and consequently more power — it gave them a sense of worth.

We do not feel safe and protected if we don't have money to provide for our loved ones, not being able to feed our family.

I helped a client of mine who was struggling with money and relationships. She was making just enough to pay her bills and most of the time living on credit cards. When we started working together, she had three credit cards fully charged, a negative bank account and still having to figure out how to pay bills to survive. She was working a lot in order to bring in income. But she was feeling ineffective, totally exhausted and empty inside of herself.

As we worked together, we could see the patterns. She was using money subconsciously as a way to avoid bigger responsibilities, as a way to run away from them, as a way to play small in life.

Funny enough, the more she was running away from responsibilities the more the universe was bringing her financial challenges so she could learn and grow. For her having more money meant more responsibilities, which was subconsciously scary. She wanted to avoid it at all cost. She always looked for a man to take care of her to avoid this responsibility. After a few years she divorced and was forced to learn by herself.

Slowly, session after session we were able to change a few of her beliefs such as: "Money is scary", "Money brings me struggle", "Money is for others", "Money brings me too many responsibilities", "I hate money", "I hate my power", "I want to be small". Have you ever felt this way?

After a few months, she was able to step up. She began feeling more in control of her life instead of giving her power away to others. She even had the courage to quit her job, move countries, find a new fulfilling job and a new partner. And she did this all by using her feminine energy and power.

Sometimes we feel we cannot escape the patterns in our life. They seem to repeat themselves endlessly. We just need to access the beliefs underneath that are running them. Patterns only happen in life for us to learn a lesson, as soon as we recognize and integrate it, they disappear.

What are Your Hidden Money Meanings?

The following exercise will help you understand what money means for you. You will be amazed at what you uncover.

Sit up straight. Prepare your mind, body and heart with five deep breaths in and out, close your eyes, while focusing on your heart.

Exercise 5: Write down all the beliefs you have around money. If you do not know an answer, ask again. Then keep asking yourself *"What else?"*

- Money is...
- Money provides me...
- People with money are...
- Rich people are…
- Wealthy people are…
- If I have money I…

Remember, write down everything that comes to mind without any kind of judgment and analysis...just continue asking yourself *"Money is...and what else?"*

If you do not identify any beliefs, just test the following ones against your own beliefs, using the Applied Kinesiology technique described on page 105.

- Money is a source of struggle
- Why earn money if it is all taken away
- Money is bad
- Money is only for others
- Money is dirty
- Money comes and goes
- Money limits me

How Rejecting Your Power Impacts Your Relationships?

By rejecting your own identity, power and gifts, you are not setting yourself as an equal in any relationships, professional or personal.

By protecting or sacrificing the feminine part of yourself, you are also neglecting parts of your gifts and not showing up authentically. In time it creates distance from people, especially close relationships. If we want others to respect us, we need to start by respecting all of ourselves.

Most of the time, we victimize ourselves by acting out our unconscious and subconscious thoughts. Then we make the other person the external guilty party. But often people are simply responding to us. It's not an easy thing to hear, but anything we encounter in life is a reflection of our own beliefs. If what we get is undesirable, it may be parts within that still need to grow and expand.

If you are not able to express your soul's truth freely, how can you expect your needs to be fulfilled? Have you stopped to reflect on this? If you express your needs authentically, other people can at least understand them, and perhaps even meet them.

But we often don't. I did this for many years. Expecting others to understand me and know my needs while I was not voicing them. As time passed, I was feeling more disconnected and unfulfilled, but still did not have the courage to express myself. Why not?

Simply because of the fear of being rejected. Funny, right? I was afraid of being rejected so I did not express my truth and wishes. As a result, I ended up rejecting myself. I created a reality I did not want and did not give people a chance to support me.

I realized that I was not in a happy place. It was only when it got too painful that I was able to react. I admitted that I created my reality. Only then was I able to take back my courage, embrace my fears and speak my truth.

It brought quite a storm in my life. There were lots of heated discussions. I had to destroy unhealthy foundations. This was extremely scary, but oh so liberating at the same time.

It is really your choice. Will you see it as life is happening ***to*** you and you are just a victim of circumstances? Or will you decide to see life happening ***for*** you and understand the lessons for growth that your experiences are providing ***to*** you?

By learning our lessons, situations rarely ever repeat themselves. And if they do, we laugh at them because we won't react the same way, and they won't even affect us. We'll have power over circumstances.

So, what is the best way to recover your voice, the free expression of your identity and your gifts? By understanding what stops you. By identifying the fears underneath your patterns around owning your own power and expressing yourself freely.

Expressing yourself freely unlocks your gifts, which allows you to create stronger and deeper relationships in your life.

What prevents you from expressing yourself freely?

Most of the time it is fear, fear of not being understood, fear of not being acknowledged, fear of not being respected, fear of not being appreciated, fear of being rejected.

But all of these fears boil down to one thing — fear of not being loved. But how can we expect someone to love us if we do not first love ourselves?

It all started in our childhood. As a child, nobody explained to us that love is infinite, limitless, and exponential, that love is unconditional, and that love is the real source of power.

We might have been afraid of upsetting our parents, interpreted as not being loved. We may have decided that a new sibling being welcomed into the family also meant losing our parents' love.

As a child, we do everything we can to catch our parents' attention, whether by being a good girl or by making mistakes to be dealt with.

We may have perceived that most of the time they are consumed by their work, which creates a belief of not being good enough to deserve their attention. Throughout our life, we replicate subconsciously those patterns. If not dealt with, the beliefs are still running in our subconscious mind.

All parents should explain to their kids that love is exponential, that they love their kids independently of what they do or say, that love is unconditional. But this is not a message that most of us get.

But let's move ahead to today. The life we have is simply ruled by the law of attraction so well described in the book, The Secret. The more you love yourself, without going into narcissistic mode, the more others will love you because you become a magnet. The more you love others, the more you receive love…the more you give, the more you get back from the universe and others.

Being aware of those patterns and beliefs is the first step towards an inner feeling of freedom as it gives us the power to change them!

The following exercise will help you understand how you hold back in your relationships, and what prevents you from being yourself.

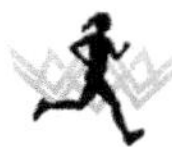 **Exercise 6**: Just reply to the below questions.

Same as in the previous exercise… Just take 5 deep breaths again, in and out, close your eyes if needed to better connect with your soul, focus on your heart to lower your brain waves and ask yourself if everything you believe is true regarding power. Once again, no judgement and analysis, just write them down... Even if you do not believe in them consciously- just write them down, everything coming up to your mind, it is your subconscious mind unlocking it for you.

What's preventing me from speaking my truth?

What's preventing me from speaking up my needs, my wishes?

What's preventing me from being myself and feeling safe with it?

When was the last time I was feeling the same? And even before that?

What was I feeling?

Who was there?

Think about a few events when you were unable to express yourself starting from your childhood? What happened? How did you feel?

Write down everything that comes to mind without any kind of judgment and analysis. Do you notice any patterns? Write them down.

So now you understand how rejecting your feminine power enormously impacts your relationship with your family, friends, colleagues, and children.

Just think about the example you want to give your kids. Will it be the example of a mum sacrificing herself and feeling empty, or of someone deeply happy and fulfilled? It was in fact the turning point for me when I realized I was not the example I wanted to showcase to my kids. I wanted them to follow the example of someone using her own voice, happiness, freedom and joy and not sacrificing it all to make someone else happy because of their own insecurities.

I wanted them to own their power as well, to determine their own life and happiness and not live in fear.

My divorce was extremely painful for all. I went through the suffering of believing I was destroying a family, destroying my kids' roots and balance, destroying their happiness.

I had to face the fears of being alone with my kids as I could not count on their father. I had to start all over again. Something inside of me was telling me I had no choice, I had to run away from this situation for my kids.... but it was also for me.

When I look back, I truly believe with all my soul it was the best decision ever, a gift from the universe. I learnt so much about myself and others. I learnt that life really happens for us, that we are supported in the process.

I really understood who I could trust or not. I deepened the few relationships I had that really counted. I had to destroy all the lies and fears inside of myself I had accepted from society. I released projections from others who preferred to stay safe instead of deciding to live.

I decided to be free no matter what and give this gift to my kids. I did it for them ultimately as my soul was dying.

Many years have passed, my kids are much more fulfilled, self-confident, positive, respecting themselves, free to express themselves, and with a different mental agility which will guide their lives.

I know many women are going through the same right now. So, my advice would be:

Embrace your fears, even love them

Hear your inner voice and

Decide to live!

Life is meant to be an abundance of love, freedom, happiness, full of joy and growth. So do not stay stuck in less than that. The universe is always here to back you up when you take the right direction!

During most of my life, I felt unsafe, unprotected, unheard, unseen and unvalued. This pushed me to numb my emotions as a way to survive and pretend everything was all right. It gave me the temporary strength to move forward.

But with this strategy, I was also rejecting my feminine essence, my sensitivity, my voice, my power, my identity, my soul. I ended up vibrating much more in my masculine energy to be able to be action driven and to feel effective. All whilst still trying to be the perfect image of a mum, of a corporate woman, wife, partner, friend. I spent years neglecting my laughter, my joy, my passion, my fulfillment.

I ended up living underneath this mask which caused me a lot of pain. After a while, I was not able to connect deeply with others as I was subconsciously protecting myself.

As explained earlier, when a woman feels unsafe and unheard, she often puts on a masculine mask, which usually depolarizes the relationship. I experienced this and many other destructive dynamics. My divorce was a loud wake up call for me. I realized I was living under layer after layer of protective masks. I had to destroy all of those to be able to rediscover who I was. It was deeply painful and scary, but the only way to recover and live.

My body was in pain and my soul was crying. But I had to find energy where I did not know I had it. I found my strength for my beautiful daughters who were also suffering.

I had beautiful friends who were there for me, listening to me, supporting me. But that alone wasn't enough. I knew the solution was inside of me and not outside. I had to rediscover my identity, my dreams, my emotions, my passions, my voice, my willingness and courage to achieve my dreams.

At that point in time, I consciously decided to respect myself, my wishes and my heart. I could not sacrifice myself to others anymore. I had to learn to speak my truth, find my inner voice and follow it, be authentic and live life for myself and not only for others! I finally felt authentic and free!

How Rejecting Your Own Power Affects Your Career?

Well, now that you've done some of the work in this book, it seems obvious, doesn't it? You are understanding the power of your feminine energy balance. How can you be fulfilled if you play small? How can you be recognized if you do not position yourself as an equal?

Anything you are running away from in your personal life, you are also going to encounter in the workplace. See it as a gift from your soul as it is usually easier to face challenges in the workplace than a divorce, or other personal problem. Even though workplace challenges can be quite painful if you are passionate and driven by growth and contribution.

I encountered many managers telling me that maybe I should "just" be a mum taking care of my kids and playing small. Clearly, they don't know how hard being a mum really is! But you can imagine the rage it created in my soul to hear this time and time again. But of course, I did not express it. Strangely enough, of course in the moment, I could not see that they were voicing my own insecurities and fears. So, I blamed them.

I also encountered managers trying to take decisions for me as if I were a child. I was told, *"This role might be too much of a stretch for you"* ,*'Remember you have kids, you should be taking care of them instead of wanting to grow in your career", "You are single, you should play smaller and stay in the background".* Often coming from an intention of caring, they somehow thought they were trying to protect me from big responsibilities. I can still feel the anger while remembering those episodes. Thinking a woman is weak and needs to be protected! Ha!

All of those events were gifts from the universe, but I didn't understand that then. I felt pushed in my emotions. I felt angry, limited, controlled. But then I began to think – why was it happening? Why was I co-creating this reality in my life? I realized I had to change something within myself first.

First of all, I had to allow my emotions to burst through the masks instead of numbing them.

Then I learned about the limiting beliefs in me co-creating this, which allowed me a space to change the beliefs of my subconscious mind and my story. And yes, I was indeed still playing small and still feeling weaker and less than others in many ways. There were many lies I kept telling myself to stay in my illusion of a safe environment, my comfort zone. The more I feel limited, the more I have the need to breakthrough.... for growth, for freedom, for self-expression.

I am still working on this now as I uncovered even more limiting beliefs as early as last week. I no longer want to feel limited as a way to push myself to breakthrough. It's exhausting and painful. As you are reading this book, I'd rather do it proactively.

It all comes from our mind, this beautiful engine designed to keep us "safe". Our mind believes the world is a dangerous place. It still believes that others want to hurt us.

If you vibrate in fear and danger...guess what? You will encounter it soon...and often. So, start by noticing your patterns, your reactions, your thoughts. Notice them with a childlike innocence – laughing about it helps you to release it and move forward.

Observing your mind with self-criticism just increases the intensity and does not help you to see clearly. Stepping back and observing your thoughts objectively is important. It helped me to see the stories and thought process I was creating.

We are all learning. I still recreate some of those patterns, but I developed a self-observing muscle and self-awareness. I just stop, smile, and acknowledge I am still learning. I look at it with humor...it makes it much less painful and brings back the child-like innocence of pure learning and growth.

I continuously work on my mindset – it is a key priority. I even do it subconsciously now. Anytime something triggers me, I ask myself, what am I feeling, why am I feeling this and when was the last time I felt it. This enables me to change my emotions, shift my reactions, and build better memories and beliefs.

Observing yourself is an extremely powerful position to be in. You can separate yourself from the events, from other's reactions and have the discernment of what is really happening, keeping your positive state and inner harmony.

Anytime I see a reaction from someone else that I do not like, I used to judge them. Instead, now I ask myself "Where am I doing this in my life? Or where am I not doing this in my life?"

Those are extremely powerful self-inquiry questions, as it brings everything back to us.

For example, I used to be triggered by people who I perceived as extremely extrovert. I saw them as "selling themselves" all around, showcasing their gifts, that they were of course driven by ego and I would think...*what a b##ch*! And I'd ask, "How could they be that way?"

But that's not the real question.

The real one is "Why was I emotionally triggered?"

I was triggered because I was not allowing myself to do the same. I could not see myself feeling comfortable doing what they did at the same level. I saw myself as quite reserved. I would not speak openly because I would feel unsafe to do so.

In reality, I was triggered for feeling frustrated with myself for not being able to speak up like them. I was afraid of others' judgment. So, in reality I was *b##ching*...myself, my own freedom of expression, not feeling free to be who I am...which is now my living incantation.

One exercise might help you find the courage to step up and embrace your fears. I did and still do this exercise with few of my clients and myself. It has the power to transform us, it has the power to give you the power back you are so afraid of. Suddenly, you see everything in your life with a different perspective.

Exercise 7: Same as in the previous exercise…Just take 5 deep breaths again, in and out, close your eyes if needed, to better connect with your soul, focus on your heart to lower your brain waves and take a blank sheet of paper.

Step 1: Imagine you are 95 years old, and you are looking back at your life.

Write down everything you are grateful for, everything you achieved, everything you regret you did not do, say or experienced.

Who is in your life, what have you achieved? How are you feeling? How were your relationships? How did your career evolve? How did it make you feel?

Start the letter with: My Dear… (your name)

And instead of using the "I" use the "You" as if you were referring to someone else and describing their life, their achievements, and regrets.

Give yourself 30 mins to 1 hour minimum, it is a profound exercise if you give yourself time to do it from your heart, just pouring words, and allowing your hands to write for you. After writing the letter, allow yourself a few minutes to re-center, to think about what you have written and how it made you feel, any concerns, any conclusions?

Step 2: You can do it just minutes later, or a few hours later. You need a friend, a partner, your children… someone really close to you *…and imagine it is your funeral, close your eyes and allow yourself to be laying on the floor, if you want to make it even more real and profound just ask your loved one to put a blank bedsheet on your body and cover your head and ask your loved one to read the letter for you.*
Step 3: Do this step right after you have heard the letter. Allow yourself to feel your emotions, they are speaking to you. *Write how you are feeling,* *What did you uncover?* *What are your new decisions?* *Are you going to drive your life the same way?* *I decide from now on to….*

I did this exercise myself 15 years ago and it was a big wake up call. I realized I was not living for myself, for my dreams, but for others. I had a huge feeling of wasting my time. I realized I was stuck with fear. It allowed me to redefine my priorities. It helped me understand my fears and love them but no longer allow them to limit me. I changed the story in my mind, telling myself that it was not fear but excitement for change that was required. I uncovered a new courage and bravery I did not know I had.

It also helps you understand the learning behind your challenges and how you can move forward in your life. This shift allows you to put your life into perspective and be the witness of it.

Now that we know how to uncover our stories, we are going to learn in the next chapter how to reframe them.

RISE UP!

TO AWAKEN THE ***SUPERPOWERS*** *IN YOU!*

Going Deeper

How Do We Access Our Subconscious Mind?

88% of what happens in our life is a projection of our subconscious mind, of our inner beliefs, fears or traumas. Our genes, the culture, the society, our family are the biggest influence on our journey, our challenges and our day to day.

The subconscious mind is like the hardware of a super-computer. Its capacity is virtually unlimited. It records all of our memories, past traumas, habits, thought forms, characteristics, self-image. It also controls all of the autonomic functions of our body, such as keeping our heart beating and breathing.

Its job is to store and retrieve data, it ensures we act the way we are programmed, based on the beliefs, memories and self-image we have stored. It does not think or reason independently. It is totally subjective.

It will co-create either flowers or weeds in the garden of our life, whichever our conscious mind has planted. That's why it is so important to be conscious of our thoughts, words and the meaning we give to situations.

It is absorbing information and co-creating your life constantly. So, imagine if your daily environment is filled with negativity, with people pushing you down. Imagine if you only think negatively, if you constantly focus on fear of something bad happening. It just co-creates it in your life. It might have already happened in your life. If you constantly think that you are fat, broke, scared of an accident.... you might co-create it.

The minute we decide to focus on something, we give it a meaning and infuse it with emotions, which dictates our inner state and ultimately the way we see life.

It all depends if you believe life happens ***to*** us or ***for*** us.

By realizing that life is a playground, to support our self-growth and that we are the co-creator of it, we also understand that we have the power of choice, the power to be responsible, the power to decide what we want to create.

By running away from any responsibility and believing life happens ***to*** us, we end up being mere victims of it, suffering the consequences of the events, of other's reactions. If this is the case, you are not taking the lead of your life neither enjoying all the possibilities it offers us.

You are negating your birth right of fulfillment and happiness and putting your life into the hands of others to decide for you. We all know deeply inside of ourselves that nobody can make us happy if we do not choose our path. Nobody has the power to make us grow if we do not choose to. Nobody is able to make us feel love if we do not feel self-inner love.

Everything starts inside our heart and not in our mind.

If we live constantly in worry in our mind, we won't be able to see the beauty of life. Living in our heart is much more powerful and fulfilling. It gives us the essential clarity to know what we need to focus on and co-create.

The meaning we give to things, situations, people's reactions defines how we see our life, how we see ourselves and what we believe we can achieve. It defines our thoughts which co-creates our lives. It is a self-fulfilling prophecy. We have the power to change it by changing the focus of our thoughts and by deciding to retrain our mind consciously.

Our subconscious mind will make us feel extremely uncomfortable, stressed and anxious each time we try to do something different or new. Its job is to keep us in the comfort zone. We have the power to reprogram our subconscious mind by taking new actions and by repeating them until they become a new and consistent behavior. That's why the fear of the unknown is so frequent and the main stopper in life. People would do anything to avoid meeting their fears, even pretending they do not have any to keep safe and in their comfort zones.

Keeping in your comfort zone is the best way to kill your creativity and future possibilities of abundance and growth.

It means that our conscious mind might tell us something that our subconscious mind does not agree with or does not recognize and might fight back. For example, I might want to try scuba diving but if I have a memory back from childhood where I was closed up in a dark room to fall asleep and super scared, I might not be able to jump in the darkness of the sea. My subconscious mind has registered that it is an extremely dangerous and unsafe situation by association.

The main goal of our mind is to keep us in our comfort zone. It has millions of years of programming; old behavior patterns whose objective was to keep us safe from any external danger. To this day, it keeps doing the same, unless we access those memories, thoughts and beliefs and change them.

Our subconscious mind has something called a homeostatic impulse, which regulates functions like body temperature, heartbeat and breathing. Through our autonomic nervous system, or homeostatic impulse, it maintains a balance among the hundreds of chemicals in our billions of cells so that our entire body functions in complete harmony most of the time.

Our brain and mind are programmed to regulate not only our physical self, but also our mental self.

Our mind is constantly filtering and bringing to our attention information and stimuli that affirms our preexisting beliefs. This is known in psychology as confirmation bias. It is also presenting us with repeated thoughts and impulses that mimic and mirror that which we've done in the past or that which we believe as true. That's why we repeat patterns over and over again in our life.

The conscious mind is estimated to be only 12% of our mind. It is the decision maker on our day to day and a word processor. It is logical and can quickly judge what is right or wrong. A quality that the subconscious mind cannot do.

What it believes and thinks might not be aligned with the subconscious mind as we saw above. You might consciously think you have no limiting beliefs regarding love, money or abundance. As for our conscious mind, it does not make sense to have restrictions. But they might be registered in our subconscious mind, otherwise we would all live a wonderful life, full of love, harmony and abundance!

Our subconscious mind has the power to reprogram our conscious mind for new behaviors and habits if we allow it and if we take action. For that we need to learn to uncover our limiting beliefs seated in our subconscious mind to be aware of them so we can change them.

We learnt to walk and talk, falling a few times but standing up again repeatedly until it became a new behavior. "Repetition is the mother of skills" as Tony Robbins says.

How Does the Belief System Work?

A belief is a feeling of absolute certainty about what something means. It is our own truth about something. A thought we have repeated endless times also becomes our own truth with time.

From 0 to 7 years old we absorb our parents' beliefs, behaviors, patterns. We are totally connected to them. We see our own identity through them. Not only do we share the same DNA, the same genetic heritage but also the same thoughts, the same behaviors, the same patterns.

It is the most influential programming period of our subconscious mind. During that time, the child's brain is recording all sensory experiences, even though they cannot speak in their first years, they can sense the environment, they feel their parents' emotions, happiness, stress, which influences their state too.

It is also a period of learning complex motor programs for eating, speech, crawling, standing, motor coordination of their hands, and later on learning advanced activities such as running, jumping, thinking.

Simultaneously, all their sensory systems are fully engaged, downloading massive amounts of information about the world and how it works.

Data from Harvard university shows that the brain forms one million neural connections every minute before the age of 3.

By observing the behavioral patterns of people in the immediate environment, primarily parents, siblings and relatives, children learn to distinguish acceptable or unacceptable social behaviors. They tend to copy them later on. That's why many children living in an abusive environment even though they have suffered with it tend to copy the same behaviors later on in their life continuing the suffering cycle even though they might feel guilty with it and judge themselves.

Perceptions acquired before the age of 7 become the fundamental subconscious programs that shape their life later on. There are no filters.

Electroencephalograms (EEG) readings show that the human brain operates at least on 5 different brain waves, each associated with a different state. They shift from state to state continuously during normal adult brain processing.

HUMAN BRAIN WAVES

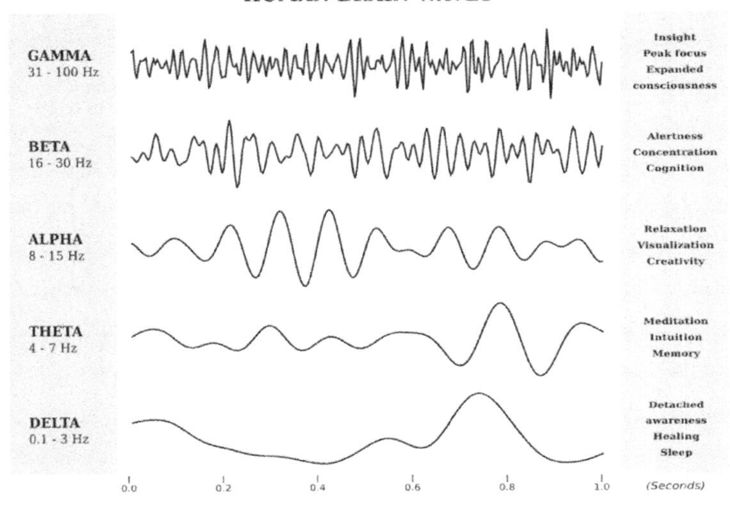

However, children's brain displays a radically different behavior; they are predominantly in delta, the lowest frequency range.

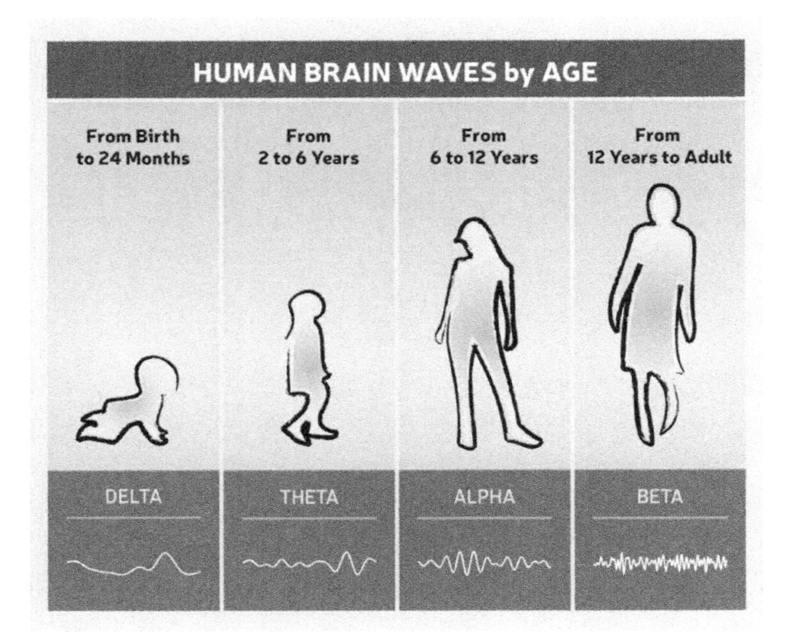

Between 2 and 6 years old, the child's brain activity ramps up and operates primarily in theta. They spend much of their time in their imaginary world and assume it as real.

By being in delta and theta, they are operating at the level below consciousness. It is a meditative state or in other words hypnotic trance. It is the same state we reach after some time in meditation. It allows us to reach our subconscious mind, understand our thought process, our beliefs.

And you might ask how can I change them?

Being aware of them is the first step towards healing and changing them. Different methodologies exist to assist you in accessing and changing them, such as neuro linguistic programming (NLP), Theta healing, hypnosis, inquiry, affirmations, incantations. I am myself a practitioner and teacher of few of the methodologies mentioned above. You can find more information on my website www.evamartins.com.

It means that during the first 7 years of their life, anything happening, their perceptions, their experiences are deeply rooted in their subconscious mind without any kind of filter. Their conscious mind is not really existent at that time and that's why it has a deep influence in their identity and behaviors later on.

Children at that age do not have the maturity and critical thinking to perceive what is right or wrong, or to decide if they accept those beliefs or not. They just assume it as their own truth, having a long-lasting impact in their life until they uncover them.

As our brain evolves, we develop our critical thinking.

As we grow, unconsciously we reproduce the beliefs and behaviors we took from others, primarily our parents and most likely what the family and the society expect from us. Get a job, get married, have kids. Often, we marry someone replicating some patterns from Dad or Mum, even though we were running away from them.

You may be doing what they expect you to do or what you believe you are supposed to do instead of what would make you happy! Sometimes you might struggle and fight against those patterns, not really understanding why you're replicating them. Not understanding why you're acting a certain way as there is no conscious reason.

Until one day you wake up feeling disconnected, unhappy, not knowing why and not knowing who you are really, if you are living your life or someone else's life.

I have done it all and felt exactly the same...

I am a second child, 3 years younger than my brother and will never forget some episodes. I was a happy joyous child, continuously singing and trying to share my happiness by dancing. I was a little chatterbox. Until the age of 3.

My brother felt threatened by me, subconsciously thinking I stole the love from our parents. In his little mind, love was limited, and I was taking part of it.

Parents almost never explain to kids that love is exponential, love is limitless. So, we almost all end up living in a place of scarcity of love, having to catch attention, needing love, sacrificing ourselves for others...none of this is true. Love is limitless, love is exponential, and the only way to open up to love and receive love is to love ourselves unconditionally. You cannot give from a place of scarcity. You cannot give what you do not have.

Between the age of 3 and 4 I was starting to own my voice and sharing it actively. I heard a few times my mum saying that I was a really bad singer, comparing my skills to my wonderful singer brother, "You are like a broken record" she would say.

If I would try to contribute to their conversation or homework they would always say "you cannot understand", "it is not for you", making me feel not smart enough. I experienced those situations repeatedly, so my subconscious mind registered "I am not good enough", "I am not smart enough", "I cannot speak out as I am not smart enough", I need to be quiet and keep my thoughts to myself". I felt constantly judged by them. Of course, it was not their intent, they were just not conscious how my brain would register those experiences. I could have reacted in many different ways.

Because I have a warrior archetype, I started to study hard proving that I was smart enough; doing everything I could to be independent and strong to subconsciously prove to them that I did not need them.

In reality, I was silently seeking their love, appreciation and approval. Meanwhile, I never spoke up, keeping my thoughts and contributions, constantly feeling judged and judging myself along the way…which brought quite a lot of anxiety.

Someone else could have reacted very differently to the same environment, accepting that they were not smart enough and having a completely different life than mine and may be playing small.

I studied the case of twin girls living in the same environment. They were dressed the same way to accentuate their similarities. They had the same upbringing, same pair of genes, and yet they had a totally different experience of life and evolved differently. All the safety environments created gave one of them self-confidence to conquer the world and she became a CEO of a large company. The other one felt disempowered, felt she could not be complete without her sister, and became depressed. She still lived with her parents at the age of 35.

Although the environment was the same, they registered different experiences and created different thoughts running their lives.

There are different stages of maturity and the ways we absorb beliefs. At a young age, we see ourselves through our parents and everything they say is taken as a given. A single source of truth, and that's the way we start our life.

Later on, as our critical mind develops, we have the power to decide if we believe in it or not, but repeated experiences have often already become reality.

After 7 years old, as kids reach primary school, they begin to separate from their caregivers by making friends. Longing for peer's acceptance and belonging, they are enlarging the scope of influence in their life, experience and environment. Their critical thinking is maturing, starting to have their own ideas, thoughts, expressing and understanding their own feelings.

The first 7 years of our life are critical in terms of creating the foundations of our mind. We acquire thought processes from our parents without a critical mind. We copy their behaviors and we take on many of their beliefs.

There are many other ways to create subconscious foundational beliefs without knowing it.

Continuously repeating the same thoughts is one way. If I continuously think that I am not good enough I end up believing in it and I will subconsciously co-create the circumstances in my life that are reflecting it.

If I believe that money is a source of struggle, then I will struggle to earn money in life, or I will struggle to keep it.

If I believe that I need to prove myself in order to be seen and recognized, then I will always attract bigger and bigger challenges in my life to be able to prove myself as it is a way to feel recognized by others.

There are different categories of beliefs. The first ones are coming from our childhood as described above. They are at the core level. Others come from our genetic background – some families tend to react the same way or do the same thing...all because of beliefs and behaviors acquired in the family genetic heritage.

We also have the collective consciousness affecting all of us subconsciously.

The collective consciousness represents all of the beliefs that you acquired from the society you live in. Each country, each society has a set of beliefs carried over and over again.

For example, at a certain age you are supposed to get a job, get married, have a baby…

In France, women would be expected to be independent, strong and feminine…

In the Netherlands, it would be expected everybody is equal…

Some other populations vibrate in scarcity, and the more they do it the more they co-create it in their environment...it is an endless vicious circle until you break it.

We also have historical beliefs based on generations and generations experiences. For example, the impact of

World War Two is still heavily present in Germany even though we might pretend it is not and ignore it.

While reading how we store our beliefs you might have memories coming to you regarding your own past. What decisions did you take based on those experiences? For example, *"I will never be like my mum"*.

You might also recognize some patterns that indicates that you have a running belief underneath. So just take few moments to reflect and do the following exercise:

 **Exercise 8:**

Think back to when you were young, less than 7 years old...

What was happening at home? What was the relationship between you and your parents? What about the relationship between them?

Did you experience love every day?

Was the environment harmonious?

Were you living in a flow of communication or silence and full of taboos?

Were you receiving the love from your parents in a way that you could really feel it? *Did you have siblings? How was your relationship with them? What were the main dynamics?* *And if you would reflect back to today, any parallel to what you have experienced in your adult life?* *Any similarities of patterns in a way you relate with others?* *Any behaviors from others in your life that you could relate to your parents or siblings?*
Focusing now after 7 years old... *How did you relate with your friends?* *How was the first day at school?* *Did the relationship with your parents and siblings change?* *How did you feel about primary school? Any special moment you remember?*

How were your first friendship' relationships? Any special memories?
Finally, after 14 years old...   *How did you live the teenage years? Any discomfort with your body changing? How did this reflect with your mood, with the relationship with others? With your parents?*   *How was the start of your career, first relationships? What age did you have your first date? What happened?*   *When did you get married or not? To who? How were the relationships? Any similar patterns with your parents or siblings?*   *Just trace back all important people in your life, whether parents, role models, some with positive impact in your life and others more challenging and see if you can recognize any similar patterns. Any identical behaviors?*

And most importantly, ask yourself, what were the positive aspects in those challenging relationships?

Anything you have to learn with them so you can move forward and not co-create them anymore?

I have done the same exercise endlessly with coaching clients, friends and on myself.

I could observe that few of my challenging managers I was co-creating in my life were the reflection of my relationship with my mother and brother. Both supporting, caring, challenging but also demanding extremely controlling, judging, non-trusting, rigid and somehow forceful.

After doing the same exercise I could understand that actually, I was learning my own inner freedom of expression, my inner spiritual power vs physical power. I was uncovering my own identity and how to put boundaries. I was learning to love myself above all, independently of any kind of judgment. The more I started to respect myself, my voice, my inner certainty and power the more I could see the beautiful lessons.

Those patterns started to disappear from my life. I was starting to attract different people in my life, leaving space for more harmony, joy and passion.
You may be thinking... **So, what can I do to identify if I have certain limiting beliefs in my subconscious mind?**

That's a wonderful question. There are many different methodologies.

One of them is to have coaching sessions with an experienced coach, who is able to identify your patterns through your words, stories, words, and experiences.

Another one is to train yourself, learn new methodologies such as Theta healing, meditation, self-inquiry and many others.

I continuously learn new methodologies and it gets easier and easier. I have trained my mind in such a way that I am able to dissociate from my thinking, observing it and identifying patterns immediately. Even though I invest heavily in training, I also work continuously with many different coaches to ensure I move forward and that I do not stay stuck in some patterns. I myself have at least 3 coaches to support me, each of them with different areas of expertise – business coaching, empowerment, NLP, intuitive.

All of this is to ensure I move forward in my life. After 20 years of practice, it is the best investment I found to do part of my self-care routine as it allows me to keep my state and clarity on what I want to achieve.

After so many years, I realized that pain and suffering are really not needed unless you believe that life needs to be a struggle and you need to challenge yourself. I realized that as soon as I identify a discomfort, I know I have something to learn and I welcome it. Then I just try to identify the lesson and change my beliefs. That is that simple!

You can learn how to connect with your subconscious mind through the theta brain waves, check your limiting beliefs in your subconscious mind with Applied Kinesiology technique. Certain meditation practices, such as Theta Healing are extremely effective, and you can reframe your brain in minutes.

Our brain is always dancing between five brain waves. They regulate everything we do, and one is always dominating at a certain point, depending on what we do. We have already touched on the delta brain waves which operate the child brain until 7 years old, here are the other ones and their impact:

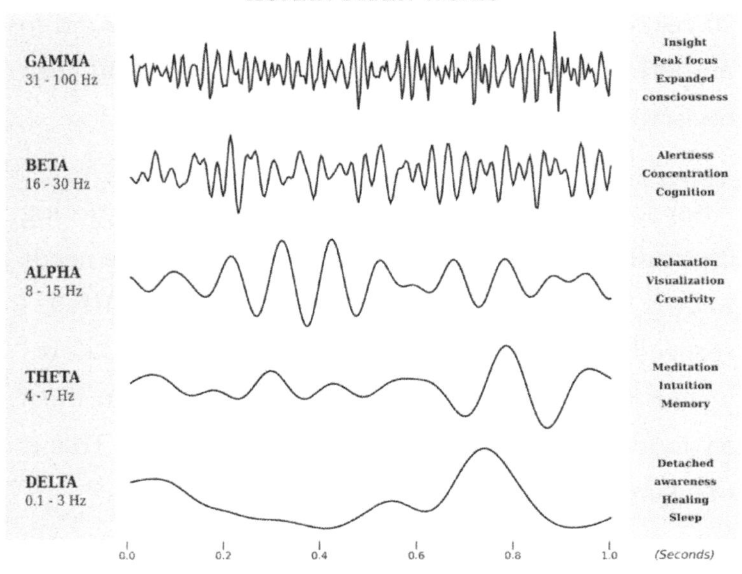

Gamma:

It is the state of learning, processing information and higher mental activity, alertness and consciousness. The gamma brainwaves cycle between 40 to 5000 cycles per second.

Beta:

We are in beta whenever we perform simple tasks such as thinking, writing, talking, or reading such as now. Beta is the state when you are alert and active, it has a frequency of 14-28 cycles per second.

Alpha:

Alpha brain waves have a frequency of 7 to 14 cycles per second. They govern the daydreaming. You are vibrating in alpha when you are in a relaxed, detached, meditative state of mind. For example, if you imagine yourself on a beach, listening to the waves caressing the sand, the birds, feeling the sun on your skin.... you are in an alpha state. It is the bridge between the conscious and subconscious mind.

Theta:

You are in theta when dreaming or in a very deep state of relaxation. It is used in hypnosis to access your subconscious mind. They have a frequency of four to seven cycles per second. When in a theta state, you are accessing your subconscious mind, your memories, sensations, deeper rooted patterns, behaviors and beliefs. Theta is the frequency of growth and change. It brings us back to our intuitive ability of self-learning.

Delta:

It is the state of deep sleep, the frequency slows down to zero to four cycles per second.

In *Theta* and *Delta,* we are operating at the level of the subconscious mind.

How Do You Understand If You Have Limiting Beliefs?

a. Let's start with your emotions

There are many ways to understand if you have limiting beliefs. The first and easiest one is through your emotions. Anytime you feel unsettled in any situation, frustrated, angry, resentful – any uncomfortable emotion would be an indication of a limiting belief. These patterns ought to be acknowledged and changed if desired.

So just try to understand what you are feeling. As achievers in life, we are programmed to numb our emotions as a way to be able to cope with situations. After a while, we might not even know anymore which kind of emotions we are feeling.

I know I have a discomfort but is it anger, frustration, sadness, stress? How many times do people ask you "how do you feel?" and you reactively say, "I am ok."

"I am ok" does not mean anything. It is not good nor bad. It is in the grey area, but do you really want to stay in the grey zone?

If not, start by identifying the language you use and reframing it. Otherwise, you are telling yourself "I am ok", without really knowing which emotions are underneath and not even acknowledging them.

Start your day by telling yourself, "I am amazing!"

And whenever someone asks you how you are, just reply, "I am awesome" and see the impact it has on you and your relationships. It puts a smile on your face and theirs.

So, the first thing is to reconnect yourself with your own emotions and body in order to understand what you are really feeling and where you feel it in your body.

Redirecting to your body helps to focus your mind and put words into feelings. Just ask yourself:

1. What am I feeling?
2. Where am I feeling it in my body?

This little easy exercise can do wonders. As soon as you objectively examine the emotions you are able to localize it, which is the first step to understanding that you are not your emotions. You are not under their control. You can see them and regain back your power to minimize them and let them go.

Emotions always bring a message. As soon as we understand it, they tend to disappear.

In the following chapter, we will continue the exercise to help you understand where these emotions come from and change the subconscious weight of the memories that have triggered them.

b. Checking Limiting Beliefs with Applied Kinesiology (AK)

The simplest way to find out whether you believe something at the subconscious level is using a simple biofeedback muscle test from the field of kinesiology.

Kinesiology is the study of how the body, and especially the muscles, move.

Nowadays, science has been able to show us that unresolved emotional conflicts, psycho-emotional trauma and limiting beliefs from early childhood and beyond remain active in our subconscious mind throughout adult life. Our limbic system (in the brain) communicates these conflicts and beliefs to our body via our autonomic nervous system (it regulates our body functions).

The limbic system is the part of the brain involved in our behavioral and emotional responses, especially when it comes to behaviors, we need for survival such as feeding, reproduction, caring for young, and fight or flight response. It supports a variety of functions including emotion, behavior, motivation, long-term memory, and olfaction. All our emotional life is largely stored in our limbic system.

The subconscious also guides our autonomic nervous system which is the part of the nervous system responsible for control of the bodily functions not consciously directed, such as breathing, the heartbeat, blood flow, organ function and digestive processes.

When there is a disconnect between what we believe as true and what we say or do, a stress response is activated in our body whether as a feeling of anxiety, fear or a physical occurrence. Responses such as feeling our stomach tightening, our face blushing…we use those triggers in kinesiology to identify those misalignments.

Here, we access the subconscious mind and understand which beliefs create a stress response. The cause of the stress might be subconscious, but the physical manifestations are captured through a weakened muscle response.

As said before, the role of the subconscious mind or autonomous nervous system is to maintain us, to keep us balanced and in harmony. So, the conflict between our subconscious mind and conscious mind triggers physical imbalances. These are stressors which results in reduced muscle strength that we can detect with muscle testing.

Applied kinesiology or muscle testing was first brought to the West by Dr. George Goodheart in 1995. Over the years it has been adopted by medical doctors, chiropractors, osteopaths, dentists, psychologists, nutritionists and others.

There are a few different ways to do the muscle testing. The easiest way to test is using the standing method, which you can do alone. I would advise to do it as a fun game to start and not take it too seriously. As you get more experienced you won't even need to do the testing as you will "feel" if the beliefs test true or not as a response in your body. To start, it is a great method to reconnect with your body instead of your mind.

First of all, ensure you are well hydrated before doing the testing as it allows your neurological system to better work.

The first step is to test your Yes and No. While standing relaxed, your arms sideways, just say Yes out loud, your body should lean forward for a positive answer, then say No, and your body should lean backwards, indicating a negative response.

And you can proceed with simple testing: My name is ... (say out loud your name) and see if you move forward or backwards, and test with a different name. If your body does not lean at all, you are likely to be dehydrated. It is always better to state your beliefs out loud as it allows you to use all of your senses.

Note that you should test in your native language as it is the language you might have used to register the memories.

You should test using positive language and avoid "don't", "isn't", "can't" and "not" as our subconscious mind does not understand negative statements and would assume them as positive.

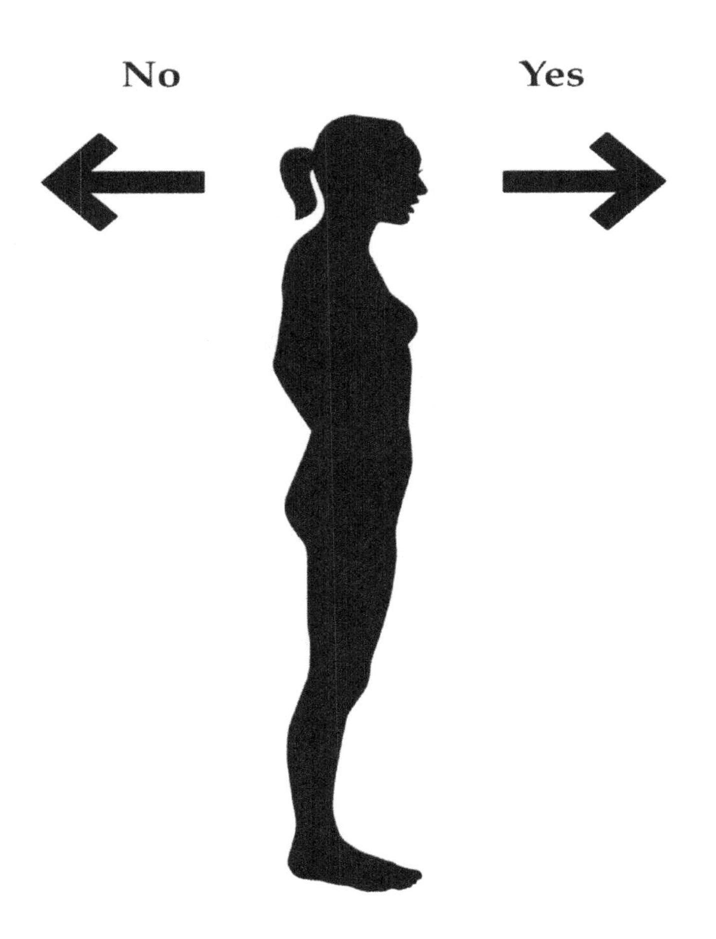
No
Yes

Another way to test is as follows:

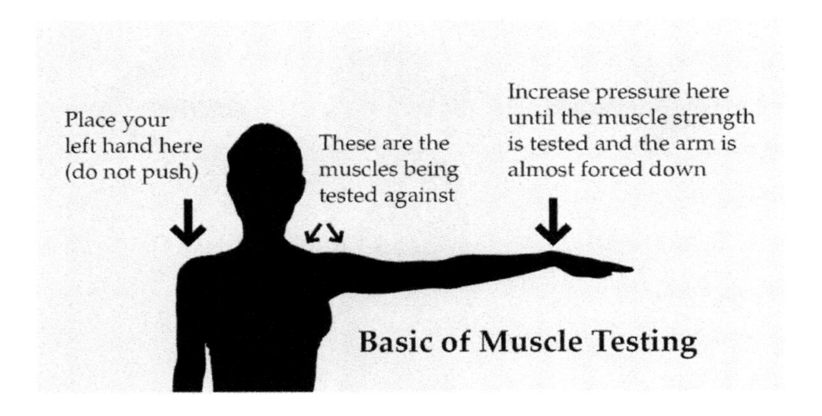

Just start by testing your Yes and No. Then you can simply state out loud your beliefs and your body will respond with a positive affirmation or negative, giving you clues if your subconscious mind believes in it or not.

In this last method, you need to say a belief as someone presses your arm down slightly and you will realize that if it is a Yes your arm will stay strong upwards but if it is a No your arm will be weakened and it will be easy for the other person to make it go down without any kind of strong pressure.

You can find many other ways online to do the muscle testing and videos explaining it. In the beginning, it is always easier to do it with someone experienced than alone.

You can find more information in the following resource: International College of Applied Kinesiology https://www.icak.com

So have fun and test the following believes:

It is safe for me to change.
Change means opportunity for me.
I thrive with change.
It is safe for me to be rich and wealthy.
I am abundant.
I can make all the money I want without effort.

Those are foundational beliefs that are empowering or disempowering you in life. Resisting change won't make it easy in life as change is a constant...

LIVE THE *LIFE OF YOUR* *DREAMS*

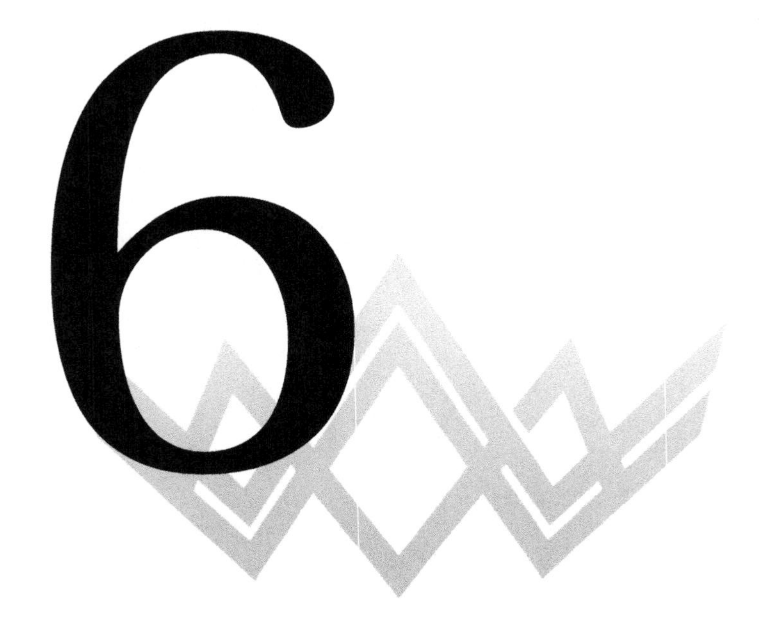

6 Taking Action

How Can

You

Help Yourself?

I am happy to share a few of the resources with you that I use. You can use those easily day to day.

One of my deepest fears is to get stuck and not grow. So, I learn everything I can to ensure I move forward in my life. Some techniques were wonderful, others not really, but they all allowed me to learn and move forward.

I am here to share with you the ones that I felt had a great impact in my life and that you can use alone. Other techniques would require that you take trainings or find a trained coach in order to better support you. I am also here for you, check out my website for more information and better understand how I can work with you. I am constantly evolving and learning new methodologies, so it is difficult to put everything here.

When I studied Quantum Physics, I understood that if you follow the science you also understand that today we can prove the impact of our thoughts in our physiology, in our life.

If we do not understand, it does not mean that it is untrue, it just tells us we may not understand it "yet".

I do not try anymore to control everything or try to have a reason for everything. The most important thing is whether I feel a positive impact on my life. It allows my brain to open to other possibilities and opportunities to grow without having to control the *'how'*, but instead focus on the impact it created.

I have a strong, curious, creative mind which loves adrenaline and self-growth so it always puts me in situations where I can challenge myself constantly.

Today, I am able to consciously manifest positive challenges and situations in my life where I can learn new methodologies instead of attracting negative events to oblige me to move forward.

I just learnt to rewire my brain. And you can too. There is no negative or positive for our subconscious mind, there are just facts. The positive or negative attribute comes from the meaning we give it.

So, if I am driven by challenge and growth, it's better to intentionally co-create the challenges I want to live to grow...

I have to say that the universe has always been here to support me in the moments I needed it the most even though I might have not seen it sometimes.

My journey started many years ago when I lost a baby. The suffering was so deep that my soul and my heart were not able to overcome the loss.

I had to let go of my mental constructs and accept that I could not control everything in life. I searched for meaning, for understanding. I was in pain and felt anger towards life. I did what I could to heal my crying soul and heal myself as my first daughter was 2 at that time and I had to take care of her and give her love while my heart was suffering. She was an angel for me at that moment, keeping my heart alive. I felt alone. I felt nobody could understand my pain.

"When the student is ready the teacher appears" ...

That's when I started my spiritual journey, trying to find answers I could not find in my heart. I met two amazing souls who became my best friends, my teachers, my mentors. They taught me Reiki and meditation. I started doing both every day and, in a few months, I became a teacher.

I still meditate every day. It became the door to my soul, to understand the dynamics in life, to understand others and my own soul. That's when I started to realize that we do co-create everything, as hard as it can be to believe.

Everything in our life is to show us back our beliefs, our thoughts, our lessons. It is a wonderful journey if we decide to take the driver's seat and be in charge of our life. Or it can be awful if we prefer to stay a poor little victim and believe we are suffering the consequences of other's acts.

I also learnt all the methodologies around the Journey from Brand Bays and Theta healing with Viana Stibal. It literally started to change my life for the better, giving me the power to choose the road I wanted to co-create. I became a practitioner and teacher as I love to go deep and share with my clients.

I also studied with Tony Robbins as a Platinum Partner and completed all of his trainings. I am a certified coach of many different methodologies (Tony Robbins, ICF...), an NLP practitioner and Master. I use Ho'oponopono, EFT, tapping.

Life is a playing field, so I test and try all the methodologies I encounter in my life and keep the ones I have personally seen a positive and quick impact. I do not believe in suffering. I do not believe we need to be in pain. So, if I can change and upgrade my mind proactively to create an impact in my life, I do it.

We have already seen in the previous chapter the AK methodologies to test your beliefs. I will share with you here easy tools to help you on the day to day to give you a quick start.

I would also encourage you to find your own teacher and coach, whether with me or someone else. I continue my journey as well, progressing in my life through more advanced training methodologies. I have a minimum of 3 different coaches on a monthly basis, all using different techniques and tool kits, depending on what I need. I am a constant student of life. Life is a playing field and I am here to play with a smile!

While I cannot teach you Theta healing, coaching and the journey methodology through a book, I would recommend finding a mentor/coach. I can definitely give you simple tools to help yourself.

If you would like to find out about working with me, please feel free to contact me at:
www.evamartins.com
www.facebook/shesgothepower
www.facebook/evemartins
www.instagram.com/shesgothepower
email: eva_martins@outlook.com
If you go to my website you will find meditations, videos and processes that can help you.

Let's start!!

Ho'oponopono

Ho'oponopono is a really simple and yet so powerful meditation or incantation you can practice.

Sometimes we think that only really complex or difficult tools are efficient but actually most of the time really simple ones are just amazing and more powerful. Ho'oponopono is one of them.

Ho'oponopono is the ancient Hawaiian secret for forgiveness.

Indigenous people living in Hawaii soon understood that holding resentments towards others is only hurting the person who is not able to forgive, creating pain and suffering.

Ho'oponopono allows us to clear the preconceptions we hold towards others.

The Hawaiian word Ho'oponopono comes from ho'o ("to make") and pono ("right"). The repetition of the word pono means "doubly right", being right with both self and others.

Ho'oponopono is a process by which we can forgive others to whom we are connected.

By healing the resentment or any other dense emotion you have towards others, you are primarily healing yourself, which makes sense. How can we be happy and balanced if we are constantly stewing over how others make us feel?

By practicing Ho'oponopono, we allow ourselves to heal the negative emotions with someone else so we can reconnect at the soul level, beyond the personality and heal any wounds in ourselves, independently of what the person did.

It brings us back to a state of inner harmony which enables us to find harmony with others as well.

We cannot change their personalities, but we have the power to change the way they made us feel and be in harmony with ourselves.

You can practice Ho'oponopono in 4 easy steps whenever you feel unbalanced through the following mantra:

I love you
I am sorry
Please forgive me
Thank you

The first step is to take responsibility over your life by taking responsibility over your emotions.

If you finally accept that you co-create your life, then there is no outer world but only your inner world and how it projects itself.

Your ego might struggle with this first step as we would fight against taking responsibility from other's wrong actions (we instead judge them). But remember we co-create everything in our life, so the first step is taking responsibility for our acts and for having co-created it in some ways from our subconscious mind. It is extremely liberating when you let go of the ego and just accept our part of the story and be sorry for it.

It is the ability to thank all of those challenges we had to face and how it allowed us to learn and grow. To look back and understand it took those challenges in order to get to where we are.

Everything has a reason to be, even though we might not understand it while facing the challenge.

Sometimes we need to go through uncomfortable situations. It gives us an opportunity to grow and move forward in life. The most powerful state you can be in life to attract everything you want is the state of gratefulness.

The more you appreciate what you have, the more you attract even more of it.

It allows you to reach a state of unconditional love. Understand that everything happens for a reason, even if it is painful. There is always a positive teaching, a lesson we take for life, which allows us to further open our heart to receive and give love.

The words are simple and powerful at the same time. It allows you to rebalance yourself and begin to view yourself differently, opening up your self-love and self-acceptance.

By applying the Ho'oponopono mantra for healing in your personal life and towards others, you find a new perspective on life, a new harmony and the release of painful emotions and conflicts.

With this inner harmony your thoughts change. Your mind becomes clearer, which allows you to co-create a change in your life. Your results change and you achieve what you truly desire in life.

To fully leverage the power of the Ho'oponopono prayer for healing into your life, I would recommend making it your morning ritual. Just take 5 minutes to repeat the 4 mantras focusing on yourself or any situation in your life. Any time you feel any discomfort, just repeat it and observe how you feel after a few minutes. Just play with it and see the results.

EFT or Tapping

EFT, also known as tapping or psychological acupressure, is rooted in the theory that when distressing emotions caused by a traumatic event are not fully processed, they become trapped in the body.

It is the trapped emotions that cause our current physical and emotional distress, not the event from the past which is over.

It is well-known nowadays that we do not remember the events, but the emotions attached to it. By clearing the emotional blockages, both emotional and physical issues can be resolved.

The "traumatic" event that can lead to the trapped emotions, can be either an emotional or physical event and can range in intensity from very subtle to life-threatening. This means that even the most subtle emotionally distressing event can have an impact on our lives until it is resolved.

The technique of tapping on acupressure points to resolve psychological issues was originally developed in the 1980's by Dr. Roger Callahan, an American psychologist who also studied Chinese medicine. Dr.

Callhan's approach is called Thought Field Therapy (TFT). Gary Craig, a student of Dr. Callahan's, developed a simplified version of TFT called EFT in 1995.

Since then, EFT has grown very quickly due to its ability to produce profound results across a wide range of issues in a relatively short amount of time as well as the fact that it is very easy to learn and use.

While still a relatively new modality, EFT Tapping has a number of research studies validating it.

The EFT Tapping procedure is a simple step-by-step process that clears the blocked emotional energy that is trapped in the body.

The process itself involves physically tapping on acupressure points while staying focused on a particular issue.

The acupressure points are connected to the same energy channels used in acupuncture.

The process of focusing on a particular issue allows the body to identify where the blocked emotions reside, while the physical tapping clears the blocked emotions. When successful, the issue is resolved to allow emotional and physical wellbeing to be restored with the ultimate result being that you feel better, happier, and more at ease.

Tapping has proven to be extremely efficient and especially in cases of anxiety and post-traumatic stress.

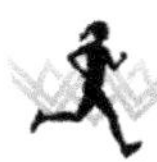 **Exercise 9**:

We can perform a session in minutes, and it is really easy, you just need to follow the following 5 steps:

1. Identify the issue

Before starting tapping I would recommend to get as clear as you can on the issue. The more specific you are, the more efficient the session and the quicker you achieve a state of balance.

For example, I might be frustrated because I am exhausted and I never stop during my day to day. I have no time for myself. I might think that I might sacrifice myself too much for others.

If I would do tapping on it, I would miss a much deeper level where it would be much more important to work with as it would have a bigger impact on your state but also all areas of your life.

In this example, I need to understand why I need to sacrifice for others. Is it because I need to be appreciated and accepted? Is it because I am afraid of being stuck and I need to feel that I am growing in life? So, it is really important to be as specific and deep as we can. You might need some help from a coach or someone else to identify the root cause.

2. Rate the initial intensity of the issue on a scale from 1 to 10

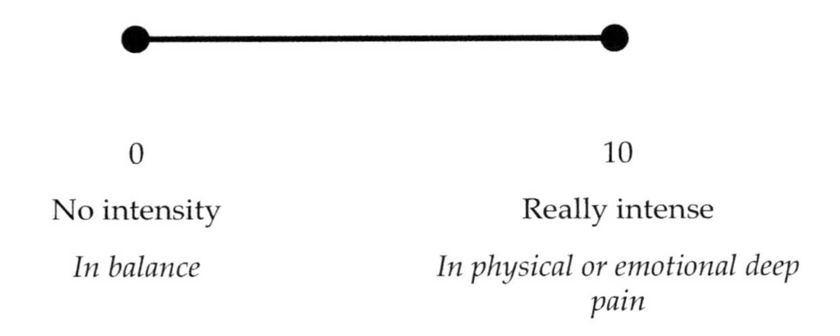

3. The set up

Before starting to tap, you need to identify your set up phrase:

"**Even though I** (fill in the blank with the issue), **I love and accept myself**"

The objective here is to focus your attention on your issue throughout the session and to accept and love yourself no matter what.

Here are few examples:

"Even though I have this fear of failure, I love and accept myself."
or
"Even though I feel stressed and anxious, I love and accept myself."
or
"Even though I feel rejected, I love and accept myself."

You should always focus on the way the problem makes you feel and not on others. For example, if you had an argument with someone you would not say, "Even though I had an argument with X"...but "Even though I felt sad with the argument I had with X, I love and accept myself." We always focus on the feeling the distress caused us.

4. Tapping sequence

The objective is to tap on 9 important body's meridian as follow:

- karate chop (KC): small intestine meridian

- top of head (TH): governing vessel
- eyebrow (EB): bladder meridian
- side of the eye (SE): gallbladder meridian
- under the eye (UE): stomach meridian
- under the nose (UN): governing vessel
- chin (Ch): central vessel
- beginning of the collarbone (CB): kidney meridian
- under the arm (UA): spleen meridian

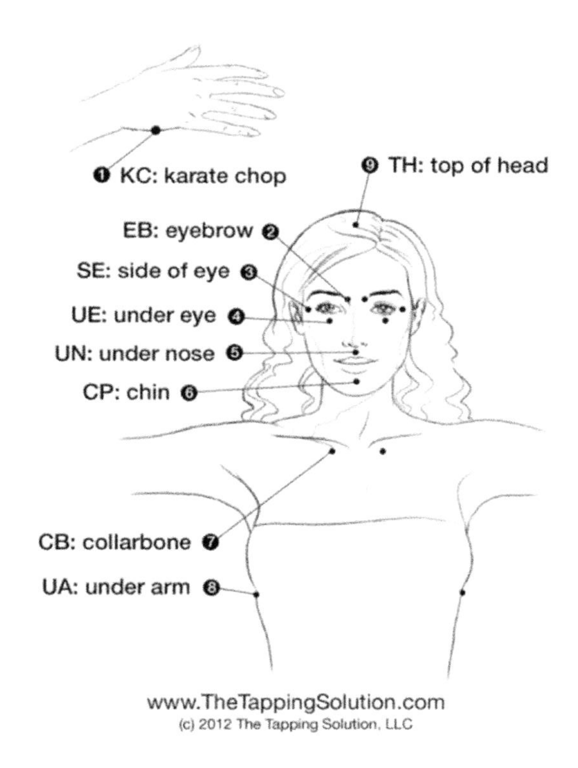

Begin by tapping the karate chop point while simultaneously reciting your setup phrase three times. Then, tap each following points seven times, moving down the body in this ascending order:

- eyebrow
- side of the eye
- under the eye
- under the nose
- chin
- beginning of the collarbone
- under the arm
- After tapping the underarm point, finish the sequence at the top of the head point.

While tapping the ascending points, recite a reminder phrase to maintain focus on your problem area.

If your setup phrase is, "Even though I feel stressed and anxious, I love and accept myself", your reminder phrase can be, "The anxiety and stress that I feel."

Repeat this phrase at each tapping point. Repeat this sequence two or three times and assess how you feel. If you still feel stressed and anxious, continue a few minutes more until the intensity decreases to between 0 to 3.

And if you have uncovered another layer, for example, sadness, or any other emotions just tap using it as well, until you feel much better.

It seems a lot but with practice, it takes a couple of minutes to feel much better and you can do it anywhere.

The Work from Byron Katie

The Work is a simple yet powerful process of inquiry that teaches you to identify and question the thoughts that cause all your suffering. It is a simple way to find your inner peace and harmony independently of your environment.

As explained repeatedly in this book, the environment where you live and the way you experience it are projections of your inner world. They are mirroring your thoughts and your beliefs which then also translates into your behaviors and actions.

The Work is a way to understand what's hurting you, and to address the cause of your problems with clarity.

Most of our suffering is based on the fact that we believe in our thoughts and we repeat them subconsciously countless times.

A thought in itself is harmless unless we believe in it, it is the meaning we give it and the emotions attached to it that are painful.

For example, if I tell myself constantly that, *I am not good enough, that what I have to say is not of value…that they will never listen to me…my kids are not grateful… my husband does not understand me…* How do you think you are going to feel when this is your focus?

You focus so much on it that you won't see anything else and you end up feeling frustrated, hurt, angry. But those feelings and the meaning you give to what is happening in your environment, is ultimately only affecting you and not others. By doing so, you are not seeing its lessons.

Instead, you end up creating a distance between you and others.

In trying to protect yourself against those feelings, you are creating deeper and more negative ones.

The Work starts by identifying those beliefs with 4 simple questions to identify the thoughts and beliefs and then turns them around to feel free of them and change your perspective.

The first step is to relax as much as you can and breathe deeply to center yourself in your heart.

Then start by writing down your thoughts, anything you believe is hurting you. Do it without any kind of self-judgment, the objective is to write as much as you can without limitations until you go to the core situation.

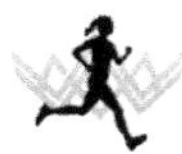

Exercise 10:

Let me guide you through the exercise with a simple example:

"I feel frustrated with my work, I feel my manager is there only for himself, he does not understand me neither wants to know about me as he is there only for self-promotion, I hate his micromanagement, I hate the fact that he does not respect anybody, I hate the fact that he does not listen to others and myself. He does not respect me and limits me"

Write as much as you can until you feel that you are reaching the core of the problem, in this case the anger comes from the fact that I am not feeling respected and feeling limited.

After we have identified the main reason, we start *The Work* with the 4 powerful questions, allowing your thoughts to come without limiting them, without judging them…for that you need to be still and true with yourself.

Let your mind ask the questions and they will surge from your subconscious mind in seconds. Write them down without any kind of judgement.

Question 1: Is this true?

Is this true that my manager does not respect me and limits me?

Yes.

Just reply with Yes or No.

If you reply with *but* or *because,* you are trying to find excuses and defend the situation. So, center yourself back and focus in your heart and how it feels and just reply what you really deeply feel. Is it a Yes or a No?

If it is a No go directly to question 3.

Question 2: Can you absolutely know that it is true?

Same as above, just reply with a Yes or a No.

Consider going deeper. Can I really know that my manager does not respect me, that he does not listen to me, that I feel limited by his behaviors? Can I ever know if he respects me?

Yes

Question 3: How do you react, what happens, when you believe this thought?

Just write down anything you feel when this happens.

"In this case…I feel frustrated, I feel angry, I feel that no matter what I would say he would anyway not listen, so I do not speak, when it is too much then I speak but I become assertive. When I feel that he is not respecting me, I just want to shout out and tell him how I feel but I do not allow myself to do it as I need to behave, he is my boss… I am angry at myself for being that loyal. I am angry at myself for not being able to speak my truth and demand respect. I am angry at myself that I am not able to impose my boundaries. I am angry at myself that I projected this situation in my life again. "Again, because it is a repeated pattern I had with my brother and mum which makes me feel I will never be free from it. It makes me feel exhausted…"

Continue your list as you witness the situation and allow yourself to be the observer. How do you feel when you believe that thought? Observe how you react and note it down.

Question 4: Who would you be without those thoughts?

This is a really powerful question. Imagine yourself in the same situation, and the other person with the same behaviors, and consider who you would be without the thought that "he does not respect me", that "he does not listen to me" …

For example, in the case above, I would imagine myself in the same situation. I would think and feel the thoughts, "my manager does not respect me", "he would not listen to me". Then I think, "who would I be if I would not believe in those thoughts?" Just close your eyes and see it happening in your mind's eye (the imagination).

Without the thoughts that he does not respect me, that he limits me and that he does not listen to me, I would see him with more clarity. I would see him smaller than he is. I would give him less power as he would appear less mature. I would understand he is trying to prove himself and be respected as well. I would understand he is just trying to seek for recognition and appreciation through feeling he is right. I would understand he is just lacking self-confidence by imposing himself to others. By seeing all of this, it feels much less impactful. I feel more compassion. I feel more powerful to say something about it in a compassionate way.

He does not want to hurt me; he just wants to be appreciated and recognized. It would not work if he would not genuinely try to respect others, he is just not respecting himself. It is not about me it is about himself. So, if I would not have those thoughts, I would feel free to contribute, I would not feel limited as he does not have the power to limit me. I do it myself…

Final step, **Turn it around**

The original statement was "*my manager does not respect me, he limits me, he does not listen to me*". When turned around it becomes "I do not respect myself, I do limit myself, I do not listen to myself."

Is this turn around true? Is it even more true than the ones above? In this situation, we would need to identify examples of *how I do not respect myself, how I do limit myself and how I do not listen to myself.*

It is extremely powerful as it reverts the situation to me and how I do this in my life.

In this situation, indeed I might see all the areas in my life where I do not respect myself, where I push my body beyond its boundaries. The way I do not always listen to my inner voice when it tells me to do something or say something - I do not listen to it nor respect it, and feel it's not even worth it, so I limit myself, I play small. It is not about my manager; it is about me and how I do not respect myself, how I do not leverage my gifts openly and safely.

We need to find at least 3 examples for each situation, genuine examples of how the turnaround is true for you in this situation.

For example, when I have a discussion with my manager, he does inquire but I do not have the courage to speak my feelings and I do not find my words to express my ideas most of the time. I feel he might not acknowledge them....in reality, I limit myself by fears of not being respected.

In this case, I would continue with a self-inquiry exercise to identify where it comes from, why I react in such a way, which are the feelings attached to it and when was the first time I felt this in my life...which leads us to the next chapter.

You can find more information and worksheet to support you at www.thework.com from Byron Kathie.

Powerful questions for Self-Inquiry

We spend a lot of time and energy trying to understand the why of certain situations. The best and quickest way is to ask yourself questions instead of figuring out the reason behind.

Our mind is trained to reply to questions.

In order to have good answers, you need to have good questions.

In this chapter, I will give you a few examples of powerful questions you can use to go deeper in yourself when you feel emotionally imbalanced but also when you feel triggered by others.

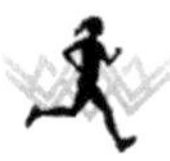 **Exercise 11:**

If we would take the example of the previous chapter where I understood that actually I limit myself, my expression by fear of not being respected or acknowledged by others.

I would ask myself the following questions:

Question 1: **What do I feel in those situations?**

Just center yourself and be honest.

I feel angry, my stomach is super tight, my throat is hurting, it wants to speak but the words do not come. I feel shaky, I judge myself, I am not strong enough…. They would not understand me…I want to run away…I feel fear all around me…and sad with myself.

It is a good idea to pull your attention to your body and try to understand how it feels as it is easier to objectively observe the feelings that way.

Question 2: **When was the first time I felt this way?**

Just ask yourself the question and wait for the memories to come. If nothing comes, just ask yourself the question again, and repeat "what else?", and "how about even earlier than that?" Just question yourself without forcing the memories. No worry – all your memories and emotions are stored in your subconscious mind. The more relaxed you are, the easiest for them to come through.

In this case, I vividly remember experiences when I was little, around 2 years old, when I interpreted that my brother was abusing his authority, as older brothers tend to do. I reacted by freezing myself. The fear was so big that I could not speak. I could not move. My brain would totally freeze like an animal feeling it would be killed any moment. I would try to numb my emotions as they would be overwhelming, and I told myself if I would express them, he would take advantage of it.

So, in reality my body still has those memories attached to those experiences and that is why I still act in the same way. In order to confirm it, I would do some AK to test a few beliefs and then release the memories, emotions and beliefs from my subconscious mind and body using NLP techniques, which would take a few minutes. It is that easy.

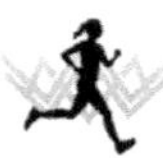 **Exercise 12**:

Oftentimes, we get frustrated with other's behaviors, with something they have said or done.

Two powerful questions allow you in seconds to see the dynamic with a different perspective.

Where am I doing it in my life or where am I not doing it in my life?

Taking an example of a client of mine. She used to be extremely triggered by her husband and especially his lack of self-care. She felt less and less attracted with time.

So, in this case we worked together and in only one session, we were able to get to the cause and release all resentments and thoughts. I just asked her "**Where are you doing this in your own life?"**

She was not expecting the question and was uncomfortable with it, which told me immediately that it was true.

She then started sharing that since she had her two kids, she gained weight. She was not feeling fulfilled anymore in her life. The only pleasure she had was eating. She started gaining weight, feeling heavy, not attractive, even feeling disgusted with herself…but of course it was too painful to feel so she was projecting those thoughts onto her own husband.

We worked on her self-love and on the dreams, she wanted to accomplish in life but that she compromised. She felt she could not have both her family and her dreams, so we worked on giving herself permission for it.

She is now a fulfilled woman. She left the marriage as it was not serving her highest and best. She lost her extra weight and felt happy again in her body independently of her weight and appearance which in turn helped her to lose even more extra kgs when she was not negatively focusing on it anymore.

In some cases, you can use the opposite question: **"Where I am not doing it in my life?"**

Taking a personal example, I used to be triggered a lot by women who would appear "too self-confident", who would speak their thoughts out loud without any kind of discomfort. I know it is quite obvious now.

In each situation, I understood I was triggered and it was nothing related to them but with myself, I just realized I was frustrated because of: not speaking when I wished I would have done it, not showing myself, hiding myself, not sharing my ideas, my thoughts, being afraid of being judged by others...not owning myself and just focusing on others. So, in reality I was not frustrated by their actions and behaviors, I was frustrated with myself for not having the courage to do it, obviously differently, my own way.... I was feeling frustrated by not feeling free to be myself.

How to identify patterns in your life

Have you ever noticed a recurring theme happening in someone else's life? In yours?

You might attract similar situations many times – same kind of people, no matter what you do you always end up without money, with people challenging your authority, or others never trusting you, betraying you…and you wonder how many times it needs to happen in your life?

We all go through the same. For a while, I was attracting manipulative people that self-described as victims of life. I ended up supporting them, giving them everything I could, sacrificing the things I would want for myself to help them…why? Simply because my subconscious mind would repeat endless programs or beliefs co-creating those situations: *money is not as important as their love, I need to put others first, I am worthless if I am not helping others, I find my significance through others appreciation…*

Our job is to identify them and update those subconscious programs to empowering ones and, in my case, I gain the awareness that the more I was sacrificing myself, trying to help them, the less I was empowering them in their self-growth. I was subconsciously trading power with love.

Well, actually it will keep happening until you learn the lesson behind the situation. Until you learn which are the beliefs running in your subconscious mind. It is not your fault; it is not the fault of others; it is just the fact that your mental software is outdated and needs to be overrun with other empowering beliefs.

As soon as you recognize the patterns and understand why it is happening and what needs to happen to change it you are free of it. It is that simple.

Situations are neither positive nor negative. The emotions and feelings depend on the meaning we give it. We gain from all of them and that is why they continue happening. In my case I was getting love or the perceived love I was trying to get…did I get love? Of course, not…as on a deeper level I was learning that I could not get love from an external source if I would not love myself first. My brain could not identify and feel love if my brain program would not know it…so I had to learn. Situations happen repeatedly for us to learn a lesson…

So, let's do a small exercise to help you.

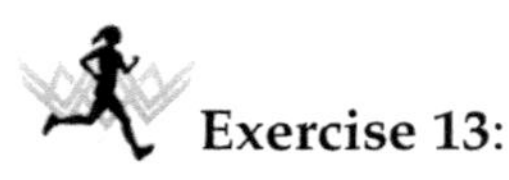 **Exercise 13**:

Same as in the previous exercise…Just take 5 deep breaths again, in and out, close your eyes if needed, to better connect with your soul, focus on your heart to lower your brain waves and take a blank sheet of paper.

Write down which are the situations that keep happening in your life. Maybe it is a relationship issue…money issue…health issue…. work issue. Just remember any of them and note them down
Write down everything that comes to mind without any kind of judgment and analysis...and if nothing comes just continue asking yourself what bothers me? And how many times it happened in my life? What happened? Which are the similarities?

And now notice the similarities…

Which are the similarities? Same dynamics in different contexts? When did it start?
Write down everything that comes to mind without any kind of judgment and analysis...

And how did it make you feel…

How was I feeling in those situations? Can you notice a pattern? Which were your thoughts? Feeling rejected? Betrayed? Abused? No power? Not understood? What did you believe was true?

Write down everything that comes to mind without any kind of judgment and analysis... for example for me in the example above I believed I had to give it all in order to be accepted and loved, that I have to put others first....just write down everything your mind is showing you as it will show you deeper patterns running in your subconscious mind

And finally, which is your gain...

Now that I have identified the patterns...why was I going through all of it? what was I trying to get from it? Any lessons? Any situation happening in our life has a gain, unless we identify it, we continue running it...

Write down everything that comes to mind without any kind of judgment and analysis. For example, for me in the example above I had to learn that love does not come from an external source but from within…

In Conclusion....

This Power

Is About You!

It Is About Unlocking
Your True Feminine
Essence

In A Way That You
Feel Free

To Be Yourself.

In summary, we are not a victim of our circumstances. Life does not happen to us but for us.

We have the choice to drive or be driven by life.

We have the choice to take the lead or be led by others and situations.

We have the choice by those simple and easy exercises to overcome situations and own our power, showcase our gifts, live a life fulfilled and connected with our loved ones.

We have the choice to free ourselves from our own self-imposed limitations and live free of them.

What is your choice? Are you going to continue allowing others to push you down?

Are you going to continue giving others your power?

Do you want to live as a victim of your circumstances for the rest of your life?

Imagine you are at the last 5 minutes of your life…and just ask yourself:

What would I feel?

Did I take all the chances I could to live fulfilled?

Did I take all the opportunities I had to make myself happy?

Did I enjoy my life?

Was I courageous enough to go for my dreams?

Who am I really?

What do I really want in my life?

If I would be truly honest with myself how do I feel?

If I would be truly honest with myself, am I fulfilled today?

So why wait for tomorrow?

You have here the chance and opportunity to regain back your life, your power and make a change in your life. If you do not do it for yourself, do it for your kids, for other women, in order to feel during the last 5 minutes of your life that you contributed to a better world…so you can leave with the realization that you did not waste your life.

My heartfelt ask here is:

STOP BELIEVING IN THE B.S. OF YOUR MIND NOW!

RISE UP!

To

AWAKEN THE SUPERPOWERS IN YOU

To

LIVE THE LIFE OF YOUR DREAMS

I love you

Eva

Extra support

If you ever feel alone, powerless, if you feel you have tried everything, and you feel stuck, I am here for you.

Feel free to contact me at:
www.evamartins.com

I have lots of free downloads, meditations, worksheets, to help you uncover your power.

And connect with our community at
www.facebook/shesgothepower
www.facebook/evemartins
www.instagram.com/shesgothepower

to get daily support from like-minded women making an impact in the world!!!

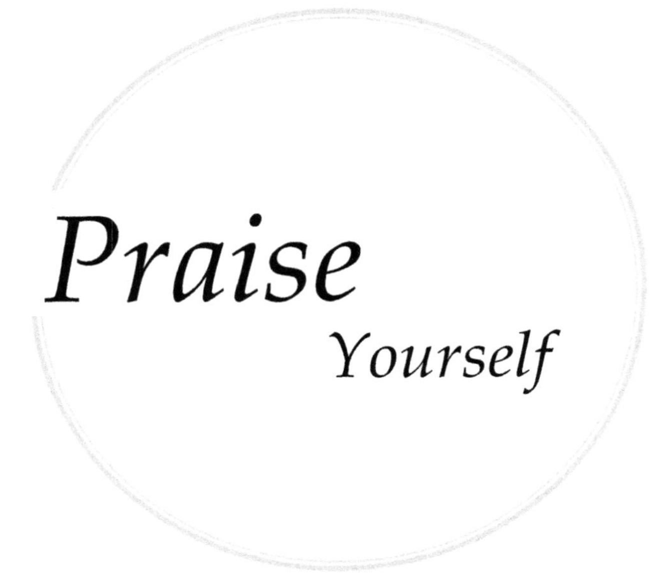

Praise Yourself

Universal beliefs to test with AK

Do not test beliefs in its negative form since the brain does not understand the word "no" or "don't". Try to always put beliefs in the positive. You might also identify dual beliefs which means that you have the positive and negative form at the same time – for example, "I am worthy" and "I am worthless". They are dual beliefs, running in your software which might bring contradictions in your life as part of you feels worthy and another part feels the opposite. It might keep you limited in certain ways. In this case we would need to replace the belief "I am worthless" and of course keep the empowering one – "I am worthy".

- I am good enough
- I am lovable
- I am loved
- I am unlovable
- I am smart enough
- Something terrible is going to happen
- The world is dangerous
- I need to control to be safe
- I am heard
- I am respected
- I can do anything right

- There is limited
- I am worthless
- I am worthy
- I hate change
- Change is painful
- I hate myself
- I need to do it right
- There is something wrong with me
- Women are weak
- Women need to obey men
- Men are leaders women are followers
- I have to work hard to succeed
- I need to be perfect
- Life is a struggle
- Life is difficult
- I cannot have it all, I need to make a choice
- I belong
- I need to belong
- I am rejected
- I need a partner to be happy
- If I have …. I will be happy
- I am a failure
- I never have time for….
- Life is unfair
- Money is bad
- Only rich people have money

- Leaders step on others to succeed
- I need to be a good girl
- I need to behave
- I reject my power
- Using my power is impacting others negatively
- My power is bad or dark
- People judge me
- Others disappoint me
- I am betrayed
- I need to make others happy to be accepted
- Women are too emotional
- I numb my emotions to succeed
- Money will make me happy
- I am too fat
- I am too thin
- I am beautiful
- I need to be perfect to succeed
- People can hurt me
- I am right
- I am wrong
- Rich people are greedy
- I am sick
- I am powerless

Feel free to test as many as you want and look at it as a game. The more fun you bring into it the easier it will be to release the negative beliefs.

By testing those beliefs, you will realize where your subconscious mind might prevent you from manifesting the life you would wish.

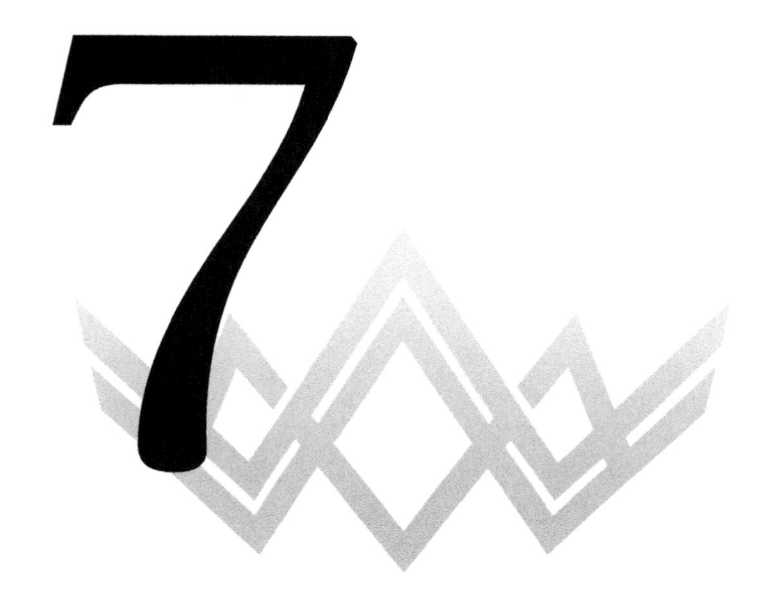

Being Inspired

Inspirational Women of the Past

Sometimes we feel alone along the journey. Culminating challenges and not feeling supported, it's easy to lose the fire inside of us. In those moments, it is important to remember we are not alone.

Thousands of women go through the same challenges and it is important to connect. Find a way to be part of a community of like-minded women where you feel valued, heard, acknowledged and with whom you can exchange ideas, solutions and feel supported.

Feel free to connect with my community through my Facebook, Instagram and website.
www.facebook/evemartins
www.facebook/shesgothepower
www.evamartins.com
IG @shesgothepower

You will find lots of tips to support you on the day to day: meditations, free exercises, online training and direct access to me. I constantly release new content to support you as we evolve with each other.

It is also important to celebrate every step we take. We are all examples for each other, for our community, for our friends, for our kids.

I would like to finish this book by remembering women that have inspired me to move forward in life, and hopefully they will inspire you too. Through their examples, I am learning about embracing my own fears. I appreciate the fears as I know their intent was to protect me, but I still move with determination towards the freedom of expression of my soul.

Throughout history, women have challenged the status quo. They fought courageously and tirelessly to be respected and treated as equals – fighting against the social norms, raising their voice, being an example of compassion, of power, of innovation, being experts in their field.

There is one thing all of the following women have in common - they are warriors, inspiring millions to also follow our calling. Nothing can stop us. We can have a ripple effect in the world. They remind us that we are not alone, that other women have paved the way for us.

Eleanor Roosevelt once challenged us all to "do one thing every day that scares you". It is the best way to continue our own growth journey. By embracing our fears, our ego, by loving it and accepting it and still moving forward we can achieve wonders like those inspiring women from the past.

Princess Diana

"I don't go by the rule book…I lead from the heart, not the head"

Lady Diana

In the early hours of 31 August 1997, Diana, Princess of Wales died in a hospital after being injured in a car crash in a road tunnel in Paris. I was there a few hours before…

I arrived home early morning after a late party night, switching on the TV while having breakfast and feeling shocked by the news, devastated…one of the women I admired the most just died.

She was one of my examples of women of power, of courage, speaking her truth, fighting for her freedom, for her fulfillment and happiness independently of the world, of judgments. Diana was a free spirit and a firm believer of equality, leading by example from a place of love. She touched the hearts of millions and still remains active in many.

She was driven by contribution, using her immense influence to empower others. She shone the light in people's lives, in forgotten causes ranging from health, and animal rights to banning landmines.

She was a revolutionary princess, not hiding behind the walls of the castle where she was living. Always going against the norms, she was constantly exposing the lies and the outdated conventions. Having the courage to defy the Queen and her husband, she exposed his wrongdoings to the world, destroying his image of a perfect son.

She was an advocate for women, and being an example, admitted her own flaws. Destroying the expectation that a princess had to be perfect, she admitted her affairs, her problems with food, her depressions and her agonizing feeling of loneliness. She was not seeking perfection like the royalty; she was seeking authenticity in a world based on social image.

To me, Diana was an example of perfection through her own imperfections, showing all of us that imperfection is actually perfect.

We are just humans going through life growth episodes, testing and learning continuously and living, despite the environment. Living despite the "norms", choosing to live life fully, authentically and free.

When I feel my courage vanishing, I remember the example of women like Lady Di who initially had a dream life, turned into a nightmare. But still having the courage to turn it around, going against her own world, deciding the dreams she wanted to live and going after them, she triumphed.

Turning the illusions of perfection into the reality of beautiful imperfection….

Marie Curie

"Nothing in life is to be feared, it is only to be understood. Now is the time to understand more, so that we may fear less"

Marie Curie

Marie Sklodowska Curie changed the world not once, but twice. She was also the first person and woman to win the Nobel prize twice and in two distinct fields, Physics and Chemistry. She discovered radioactivity and named it as such. When World War I broke, being committed to support and share her abilities, Marie Curie helped to develop portable x-rays so that soldiers could be examined on the field. She drove the ambulances herself to the front lines during the war.

I can only imagine what Marie Curie went through. Being a scientist myself, I started my career in a men's world where the place for women was limited. We felt we were the exception and most of the time had to act as a man just to be heard...I am not even speaking of being accepted. It is another story.

Marie Curie was a pioneer, a trail blazer and a role model for women, definitely for me. If she could make it in a period where women were not even expected to study, then I could also achieve my dreams and embrace my courage. She was fighting against gender stereotypes, which was not even considered at that time.

Marie Curie challenged the collective consciousness at a time where women's only "choice" was to stay home to take care of children and the house. She decided a different career path, following her father's steps into science by studying mathematics and physics. This was totally unheard and unacceptable in the 19th century.

She taught me that with determination, passion and courage I could defy the established norms and be an example for others.

She was determined, courageous, driven by growth and contribution and wanted to use science to have an impact in the world. She was intelligent, a woman of action, adventurous and brave to take these first steps in a man's world.

As you can imagine the challenge was not small…

Born in Poland on November 7, 1867, she was the youngest of 5 children. She attempted to join the university in Warsaw but was rejected for being a woman. Determined as she was, she did not give up and joined a "floating university", an underground educational system that moved from location to location to avoid being discovered, and studied physics, mathematics and chemistry.

In 1891 Curie moved to Paris, penniless, to continue her scientific studies on radioactivity at the Sorbonne University. Studying during the day and tutoring in the evening to pay her bills. Later on, she met her husband Pierre Curie, and went on making amazing discoveries on x-rays and two new elements radium and polonium, using her husband's laboratory equipment.

After his sudden death in a car accident, she took over his lab as well his own classes, being the first woman to teach at the prestigious University of Sorbonne.

She never questioned the possibilities that stood before her and just grabbed them.

She not only inspired the scientific community with her research and discoveries, but she also taught women to go for their passions, to not step back just because the environment is not ready yet...she just made it happen.

All of her life has been a testimonial for feminine power, for strength, teaching us we can manifest our dreams.

She challenged the typical social feminine and masculine roles, fought against the accepted and unspoken norms…an inspiration!

She taught me that independently of the norms or the environment, we can always go for our dreams. With passion and determination, we always make them happen.

By remembering the challenges other women went through, we are able to minimize the impact we give to our inner stories, dramas, fears, and inner lies. They all appear quite small compared to the roadblocks Marie Curie had to overcome.

Being a scientist myself, having studied Pharmacy, Chemistry and Quantum Physics, she is one of my role models for courage, determination, growth and passion.

Rosa Parks

"I have learned over the years that when one's mind is made up, this diminishes fear; knowing what must be done does away with fear."

Rosa Parks

Rosa Louise McCauley Parks was born in Alabama, on February 4th, 1913 to Leona, a teacher and James, a carpenter. She was little when her parents separated and moved with her mom to Montgomery.

She lived in a period where laws dictated that African Americans had to sit at the back of the bus while white people sat in the front. If the white section became full, African Americans had to give up their seats in the back for whites.

One day Rosa refused…she refused to give up her own humanity, her own life, her own rights, her own values. It was fundamentally wrong, and she was no longer going to allow it.

Rosa Parks further ignited the civil rights movement in the United States by refusing to give up her seat to a white man on that Montgomery, Alabama bus in 1955.

She was arrested for her defiance, but she persisted, challenging the segregation order in court.

Her action inspired the black community in their fight for their rights, to be respected, to have a voice.

Her story inspired me, reminding me that despite the environment we are allowed to have a voice, we are allowed to exist equally.

From a young age, I believed women were weaker until I heard stories about women like Rosa Parks who defied the conventional. For many years, I've wanted to work for "Médecins sans Frontières MSF", to travel the world helping minorities, supporting young girls in their studies, raising my voice for women respect and gender equality. This is still a dream of mine...and I know it is possible. And this book is part of this dream coming true.

Rosa Parks inspired not only the local black community to organize the Montgomery Bus Boycott, but also showed women they had power! The boycott lasted more than a year, led by the young activist Rev. Dr. Martin Luther King Jr.

Rosa Parks, recognized as the mother of the civil rights movement, became a symbol of strength and dignity inspiring millions to fight for their rights independently of the color of their skin. She was a quiet, humble, charismatic leader, sacrificing herself for the needs of others.

Rosa Parks never felt ashamed of the color of her skin, nor of her femininity.

She led by example, believing that her acts would speak louder than her words, setting up a new standard. Inspiring others by showing the example to do the same instead of loud speeches, battling or aggressive actions. She was a lady, a symbol for human rights and feminine power and bravery. She is for me a role model of what leadership really is and how we can inspire a team, and a community to better serve the population.

Mother Teresa

"Be faithful in small things because it is in them that your strength lies."

Mother Teresa

Mother Teresa lived a life of love, charity and compassion in a world that valued prosperity and ambition.

Born as Anjeze Gonxhe Bojaxhiu, August 27th, 1910, in the town of Skopje, Yugoslavia, she was also called the 'Angel of Mercy'. At the age of 18 she left home to join the sisters of Loreto, a group of nuns in Ireland. A year later she moved to India and taught at a Catholic school for girls.

In 1950 she received Vatican approval to create the Missionary of Charity, a group of religious sisters who took the vows of chastity, poverty, obedience and to dedicate their lives to the "poorest of the poor". The Missionary still exists and counts more than 4000 nuns today.

Throughout her life, she received more than 200 prestigious awards and honors, including the Nobel Peace Prize in 1979.

Mother Teresa was a missionary and Roman Catholic nun who dedicated her life to helping others. She was convinced that each human is called upon to do something bigger than themselves, serving the common good of all. For her, it meant feeding the poor, teaching kids in the streets in India, providing care for the sick and providing shelter for the homeless. She could see beauty in all individuals who were abandoned or rejected by the society. Stripped of all earthly desires, she carried love in her heart. She could see the soul of each and every individual instead of their appearance.

We often forget that we are all humans with our own fears, beliefs, experiences...we get stuck in our own stories or realities.

Mother Teresa taught me to see the soul beyond the personalities, and to see the challenges we all go through. She taught me how to be compassionate and have empathy towards each other. She also reminds us that our problems are so insignificant when you compare them to those that do not have a shelter to sleep in, or food to eat, or no one to take care of them.

She was a little woman of five feet who conquered the hearts of millions in a big way with her determination, love, acts, compassion and messages. She travelled the world to raise the awareness of imbalances, forcing the world to re-examine their own priorities, hearts and minds. She challenged the status quo. She met presidents, princesses, queens…always fighting for her cause, for the poor. It was impossible to say no to her when she wanted something.

Her devotion in helping others was bigger than herself, bigger than any fears she might have had.

She taught us that it is the goodness, kindness, unconditional love and selflessness that resides in every human heart that defines us, not our successes. It is the impact that we bring to other's lives through love that defines us, not what we achieve or conquer. She shocked the world with her messages, in devoting herself to the poor and those rejected by society - the lepers, the sick, the homeless.

She was strong and feminine, she was power and sensitive, she was love and action-driven… a true example of feminine power having a huge impact at a global scale and in the hearts of millions.

She believed the biggest problem on earth was people being unloved; so even in her exhaustion, if all she could offer someone was a smile, she gave it.

It is not about getting - it is about being, it is about giving a smile to others. It is about who we become in life.

Eva, inspired by Mother Teresa

Cleopatra

"I will not be triumphed over."

Cleopatra

Cleopatra reigned as a queen of Egypt during the 1st century. She is one of the most famous female rulers in history and a prototype of the romantic *Femme Fatale*.

Cleopatra VII Thea Philopator ("Cleopatra the Father-loving Goddess"), born in 69 BC, daughter of the king Ptolemy XII. Cleopatra VII was part of the Macedonian dynasty that took overrule of Egypt in the late 4th century B.C.

She shared the throne at 18 years old with her brother, who was much younger, when her dad died. It is likely that the two married soon after their dad died.

She is well known for her beauty, but even more for the divine feminine energy she incarnated, knowing how to use it for her advantage. She knew the power of her femininity and did not shy away from using it like a goddess to get what she wanted. She used it in charming Julius Cesar to gain his protection, and in marrying Mark Antony.

She was the personification of elegance and confidence, smart and astute. She carried an air of sensuality and wisdom. She knew that being feminine was not a weakness but a power she played with, all her life. She knew her sensuality, smartness and confidence were her strengths.

It was not all about her beauty or sensuality - she knew she had to also be as smart as men. She spoke many languages, was educated in philosophy, mathematics and astronomy and was greatly respected for it.

The combination of owning and mastering her femininity, with her smartness and knowledge made her super powerful - and she knew it.

Cleopatra left behind a beautiful example of a feminine leader in a male dominated society, at a time where Egypt was struggling in internal and external conflicts. She proved to be a really strong sensitive leader at the level of her masculine counterparts.

When in doubt, or in fear I remind myself of the stories and achievements of these powerful, feminine women. I remind myself to speak up and move towards my inner freedom like Lady Di, or stay true to my values like Rosa Parks, be compassionate and caring like Mother Teresa, go for my dreams like Marie

Curie....and own my power and femininity like Cleopatra. They all lived in a period when women were not supposed to have rights, a voice or choices but they all broke their own glass ceiling, becoming an example for millions.

They did it - so can we!!

Printed in Great Britain
by Amazon